The Thalidomide Catastrophe

How it happened, who was responsible and why the search for justice continues after more than six decades

Martin Johnson, Raymond G. Stokes, Tobias Arndt

Onwards and Upwards Publishers
3 Radfords Turf
Cranbrook
Exeter,
EX5 7DX
United Kingdom
www.onwardsandupwards.org

This first edition is published in the United Kingdom by Onwards and Upwards Publishers (2018).

ISBN: 978-1-78815-629-5
Typeface: Sabon LT
Graphic design: LM Graphic Design

Printed in the United Kingdom.

PUBLISHER'S NOTE

The views expressed in this book are those of the authors and do not necessarily represent or reflect the views of Onwards and Upwards Publishers.

Acknowledgements

This book has been produced with help from a vast number of people, both those within the worldwide thalidomide "community" – survivors, those affected by the drug – and those who only first engaged with the subject during the time we were working. The authors are grateful to all who have helped in any way. The Thalidomide Society (UK) is the organisation which provided the main foundation for the work, with its invitation to present the early material during their meetings in 2010 and 2011, but especially at the 50th anniversary event in London, on 26 May 2012. The presentation delivered on that occasion was the basis for chapter one. The Contergan Society of North Rhine-Westphalia was another body providing much information and encouragement. Support from Contergan (thalidomide) survivors in Germany has been very strong, and the first public airing of the authors' argument that the thalidomide drug was most probably not invented at Chemie Grünenthal GmbH was at a combined meeting of the German Contergan Societies in Berlin, on 26 November 2011. In addition, there has been the support from virtually all the thalidomide organisations representing survivors around the world, including FfdN of Sweden, TVAC of Canada, the Ishizue foundation of Japan, and the societies representing Australia, Austria, Belgium, Brazil, Ireland, Italy, the Netherlands, Norway and Spain.

Individuals who have helped with testimonies and historical and other information include thalidomide survivors Monika Eisenberg-Geginat, Bjorn Håkansson, Claudia and Udo Schmidt-Herterich, Andrea Kornak, Mercedes Benegbi, Shoshana Duizend-Jensen, Leigh Gath, Fred Dove and Phil Williams. Parents of thalidomide children giving new evidence include Michael Carr-Jones and Sadie Galvin. Michael Howard, a former 'T-Force' officer, directed us to the organisation's post-war debriefs of German scientists held at Duxford. We are also grateful for information and encouragement supplied by the former *Sunday Times* journalists Bruce Page and Sir Harry Evans; supporter Jonathan Stone; and researchers Inge Mecke and Ruth Ziegler.

Assisting the project in different ways were thalidomiders Geoff Adams-Spink, Nick Dobrik, Guy Tweedy, Craig Millward, Rowland Bareham, Stevie Sinclair and Wendy Tomes, together with several other members of the thalidomide campaign group and the Thalidomide Trust's National Advisory Council; also Thalidomide Trust chairs Sir Michael Wright and Sir Robert Nelson with the support of the other trustees.

For help with the medical and scientific aspects of the work, we wish to thank Drs. Claus G.H. Newman, Janet McCredie, Harald Mückter, Elizabeth Horak, Tosca Kinchelow-Schmidt, E. Clive Joseph and Professor David Healy.

The work has involved a considerable amount of archival research, and we wish to thank the staff of the following archives for their considerable help: Imperial War Museum, Duxford, Cambridgeshire (UK), the Bundesarchiv (German Federal Archives) at Koblenz and Berlin (DE), the Landesarchiv NRW, Duisburg (DE) and the Archiv der Sozialen Demokratie, Bonn (DE).

We have been particularly grateful to Dr. Ruth Blue (Thalidomide Society) in her efforts to track down people prepared to supply their personal photographs, and to all those individuals themselves. Trevor Beattie of BMB has generously provided his time and talents in creating our cover design and some of the graphics used inside.

This work has taken more than eight years to bring to completion, and it is possible we may have not included everyone who has helped. If we have overlooked anyone, we ask their forgiveness, and trust that the accuracy and importance of the narrative will be what matters.

Martin Johnson, Raymond G. Stokes, Tobias Arndt
Saint Ives, Glasgow and Brussels
October 2017

Contents

Foreword by Sir Harold Evans

I could never forget the brave sweet innocence of the infants at Chailey Heritage hospital and school in Sussex. The youngest in 1962 were only three, attempting to navigate a strange new world with their limbs foreshortened, short shoulder flippers instead of arms, toes from their hips, or no limbs at all. They were a few among the thousands of infants worldwide attacked in the womb by the poisonous pill we know as thalidomide. It was patented in 1954 by Chemie Grünenthal, the German company headed by Hermann Wirtz (1896-1973) and his family in the Rhineland town of Stolberg. Hermann's firm had prospered as part of the Dalli Group in the Nazi era, making soap and detergents for the Wehrmacht; Aryanisation enabled them to take over Jewish businesses for little money, forced and slave labour was on tap. Postwar, with high demand for penicillin, they tried their hand at pharmaceuticals. They patented their thalidomide compound as 'Contergan', promoted it as non-toxic, no side effects, completely non-poisonous and completely safe, better than all other tranquillizers for relief in pregnancy from morning sickness and sleeplessness. They licensed it in 79 countries under no fewer than 49 different brand names.

Every one of them was a lie.

This momentous book, teeming with revelations, is the first comprehensive history of thalidomide. It takes us from its murky origins in the Nazi era to the shadows behind its fateful move into pharmaceuticals, Wirtz's conduct in the catastrophe, and his astounding escape in his criminal trial. The three authors came together one by one – I think of them as three gallant Musketeers. Martin Johnson was for 21 years a pilot in the Royal Air Force, before flying high as the director of the UK Thalidomide Trust in 2000, navigating so well the survivors have an average income of £50,000 a year. Tobias Arndt, an unstoppable researcher, was moved to offer his services to Johnson and the UK thalidomide campaigners after seeing the moving German documentary 'Eine einzige Tablette' ('Just a single tablet'). And Johnson recruited as the third Musketeer the renowned historian of IG Farben,

Professor Raymond G. Stokes, at the Centre for Business History in Scotland at the University of Glasgow.

I salute them. I have written extensively on thalidomide, along with my *Sunday Times* colleagues in the seventies. In January 1973, with allies in Parliament, thalidomide families and the City, we finally won compensation ten times the dismissive offer made by the whisky bottlers Distillers, who marketed thalidomide as Distaval under licence. Three and a half years later, the European Court of Human Rights freed us to publish our investigations on the causes of the disaster suppressed by the British government. In 1979 we published the Insight Team's *Suffer the Children: The Story of Thalidomide,* subsequently the basis for the documentary, 'Attacking the Devil', by Jacqui and David Morris (on Netflix).

From 1959 to withdrawal of the pill in November 1961, the shock of tragic births in Britain and Europe and Canada and Australia was intense, but the following decades were marked by a series of aftershocks. Heedless national governments inflicted further cruelties on the distraught families, abandoning them and their afflicted children to the mercies of a powerful corporation. Chemie Grünenthal and Distillers and the rest of them didn't have to worry about how to cope with the traumas of an armless, legless, or deaf, blind, incontinent, sobbing child, as mothers did for a whole ten years or so, waiting for some paltry settlement pronounced, if they got that far, by a judge who had no idea how to assess the lifetime actuarial needs. In Britain, the government rejected a fact-finding public inquiry of the kind that attends an air or train crash and then, in the person of the Minister of Health, Enoch Powell, sided with the perpetrators of the disaster. All the mainstream press went along with the notion the tragedy was an act of God rather than sloppy science multiplied by greed. Some countries were so lax they let the pill linger in the market months after its official withdrawal. The 180 Spanish victims in their Avite campaign won in the lower court, and then were appallingly ruled out-of-time by Spain's reactionary Supreme Court. Justice was corrupted, most foully in Germany where Chemie Grünenthal to this day keeps saying it did the standard tests of the time when it plainly did not.

The Thalidomide Catastrophe takes the story deeper and further. It credibly estimates the total number of deaths and demonstrates how many thousands of victims, both those who survived and those who died, could have been spared very late in the day if Chemie Grünenthal had taken any notice of the early alarms; they did the contrary. They suppressed them. And the toxic pill sold by Chemie Grünenthal and its licencees is still damaging babies in the womb in many parts of the Third World. At the half century, at last, the book reports significant progress, gathering force from 2005 in a perfect storm: new lawsuits; unceasing efforts in Europe from the UK thalidomiders; the awakening moral sense of the legal successors to the key licensees, Distillers in the UK and Astra in Sweden; funding commitments by the governments of Germany, the UK, Italy, Austria, Canada, Brazil and Belgium; the 2008 creation of the International Contergan Thalidomide Alliance (ICTA); the 2013 class action triumph of Peter Gordon's law firm for thalidomiders in Australia and New Zealand; editor David Walmsley's rapid success at *The Globe and Mail* in Canada in 2014. And at last in Britain there was a Minister of Health who had a soul and a spine to go with it. Labour's Mike O'Brien rose on the floor of the Commons in 2010 to deliver a full and unconditional apology.

The Thalidomide Catastrophe carries conviction by its scientific rigor, its energy in tracking evidence, its restraint in reaching conclusions and the cool clarity of the writing. Pause to imagine the resonance of one concise paragraph:

"The most severely damaged survivors have four-limb damage and are blind, with various forms of brain damage. This was the almost inevitable result if a mother took a tablet each day from around the 20th to the 30th day after conception. A tablet on days 21-22 could result in loss of, or damage to, the eyes. For days 22-23, intake of thalidomide could result in similar damage to the ears and face, whereas one tablet on day 24 could result in a complete absence of arms, and on day 29 an absence of legs. It is likely that the most severely damaged survivors were a tiny fraction of those living through such trauma; the majority damaged to this degree could not."

Upwards of 100,000 babies were destroyed. Between 40% and 45% of the 25,000 thalidomide babies born alive died before their first birthdays. Kevin Donnellon, we read, was a four-limb damaged baby, not breathing, shoved out of sight in a box under the delivery bed to spare the mother. "The doctor inadvertently kicked the box, and the baby started crying and survives to this day. Kevin went on to achieve an education to postgraduate level, become a university lecturer, a campaigner against cruise missiles and a father." But thalidomide's effect was not confined to pregnant women. From its very early days men and women who ingested it as an over-the-counter sedative were diagnosed with polyneuritis, the painful and incapacitating nerve damage. Chemie Grünenthal knew all about these affects in 1956 before bringing the drug to market. They took no notice. As the drumbeat of complaints began to rise, they feigned ignorance – "first we ever heard of that" – and then passed them off as temporary, or allergies, statements punctuated by outright lies.

The death camps

The Musketeers grapple in fascinating detail with the central questions: Did the drug originate in the Nazi death camps? Was the tragedy preventable? Precisely how many did thalidomide kill and maim? What was the role of the German federal government in the criminal trial of Grünenthal executives?

It's exhilarating to see how they follow up a lead. In October 2008, at a meeting of the Thalidomide Trust, the medical adviser asked "an apparently straightforward question that does not seem to have occurred to anyone previously": How did the authors of the patent specification know the detailed information contained in it about the effects of the drug on humans?

The point is that the information derived from the testing was undertaken only *after* the patent was filed. So where had it come from? The suspicion naturally arises that it might have been from experiments on humans in the concentration camps, an appalling thought, and one of the most impressive features of *The Thalidomide Catastrophe* is how the writers refuse to jump to conclusions. They take the reader through all the evidence they have accumulated, weigh it carefully, and suggest various scenarios. How significant is it, would you say, that Grünenthal was not able to produce the animal test records? (Sorry, said the scientific chief, Dr. Heinrich Muckter, we lost them all in a move.) Is it a coincidence that Distillers in the UK using the patent information could not replicate the result? On a tip from one of the surviving members of the T-force that entered Germany as the war was ending, the Musketeers scurried off to a Battle of Britain airfield at Duxford, in Cambridgeshire, where the Imperial War Museum had converted a former NAAFI club into a storeroom. The reports of the Combined [British and American] Intelligence Objectives Subcommittee (CIOS) revealed a lot about scientists who had been connected with

Grünenthal, and the range of compounds that were similar in nature and effects to thalidomide. Mückter at the Army Institute for Typhus and Virus Research in Kraków fatally tested various drugs on scores of inmates at Buchenwald. Otto Ambros of Auschwitz watched concentration camp prisoners die from experimental gas. And the Duxford boxes revealed that Mückter's mentor, Professor Werner Schulemann, had synthesised various phthalimide compounds, at least one of which (an attempt to combine a barbiturate molecule with a phthalimide) had "a nearly identical composition and structure to thalidomide itself".

The Musketeers' careful evaluation of the strands leads to the conclusion that there was "a strong likelihood" that thalidomide was developed outside of Chemie Grünenthal, and probably also before 1954, the misleading year in the Grünenthal mythology. The Musketeers concede that "It is even possible" that thalidomide was developed during the Nazi period. They don't feel able to nail that as firm and fast, but when you read the description of the networks of individuals and organizations involved in thalidomide, you see the behaviours established during the Nazi period. After all the Musketeers' scholarly step-by-step qualifications in scrutiny of the evidence, it's a relief to reach a resounding judgment on the trio of Schulemann, Mückter and Ambros: "Participation in and (at the very least) tacit acceptance of murder, enslavement and human experiments formed part of their shared CVs. In the pursuit of medical, scientific and technological excellence and commercial gain, these men and the many like-minded individuals around them demonstrated a complete disregard for normal human values, and attained what they eventually achieved only at the cost of wreaking havoc and extreme suffering. The disastrous consequences of this pattern of behaviour became evident in the thalidomide catastrophe, which featured the firm Chemie Grünenthal at its heart."

The sham trial

The mystery of the tests on humans might have been resolved at the criminal trial. The North Rhine Westphalia prosecutors accused nine Grünenthal employees with committing bodily harm and involuntary manslaughter. The bill of indictment ran to 972 pages with 351 witnesses called in support, 29 technical experts, and the trial was estimated to take at least three years. It opened in the pretty town of Alsdorf, near Aachen, on 27 May 1968. It was shut down on 18 December 1970.

The judges did not convict the company, nor exonerate it. They simply freed the nine accused, granted Grünenthal immunity from any further criminal proceedings, and imposed silence on the 2,554 German families who had no choice but to go along with a miserable compensation scheme contrived by the government and the company (valued at only ten per cent of the claims).

The Thalidomide Catastrophe is unsparing in condemning this bizarre result and the stealth by which it was realized. While the witnesses testified and endured cross-examination in noisy, angry scenes in the courthouse, Grünenthal directors and their lawyers began meeting in secret with the federal Health Ministry – without families or their representatives. And for good measure, during the trial the prosecution became the ultimate responsibility of one Joseph Neuberger, appointed Justice Minister of NRW, who just happened to be the defence attorney for Hermann Wirtz. Readers can make their own judgments of the official German state and federal denials and obfuscations that have followed the archival revelations produced by the Musketeers. There is no doubt in my mind. Fifty years after the deaths and sufferings the thalidomide tragedy is marked not by the final celebration of justice, but the odour of corruption and cover up.

The political leaders and officials who continue to deny the colossal cover up at the Alsdorf trial risk putting themselves in proximity to the odious Holocaust deniers. Germany has earned its high international esteem by its honourable recognition and repudiation of the crimes committed in the nation's name. The nightmare of thalidomide would best be ended by the appointment of five international jurists charged not with criminal adjudication but with truth.

The infants at Chailey and their companions deserve nothing less.

Sir Harold Evans, former editor of *The Sunday Times* and *The Times,* is editor at large at Reuters; his views are his own. He is the author of *The American Century; They Made America; My Paper Chase;* and *Do I Make Myself Clear?* and co-author of *Suffer the Children* with Philip Knightley, Bruce Page, Elaine Potter and Marjorie Wallace.

Introduction

ON 18 DECEMBER 1970, THE JUDGES presiding over the criminal trial of executives of Chemie Grünenthal, the company that developed and marketed thalidomide, announced their decision to suspend what by then counted as the longest-running legal proceeding in German history.[1] The result was anticlimactic in the extreme. After six years of investigations that had preceded the start of the trial, followed by more than two-and-a-half years in court, the judges suspended proceedings without a final verdict on who bears criminal responsibility for the thalidomide disaster: the defendants were neither exonerated nor found guilty. And from that point to the present, the company has never shouldered any real responsibility – criminal or otherwise – for causing the massive devastation that the drug inflicted. Introduced as an allegedly safe hypnotic sedative, it soon was widely used for the treatment of morning sickness before its capability for causing birth defects and infant deaths led to a worldwide catastrophe.

As a result, and quite understandably, there is a sense of justice denied among the catastrophe's victims, who include not only large numbers of often severely disabled survivors and their families, but also the families of the thousands of babies who were stillborn as a direct result of their mothers' use of the drug during pregnancy. Events and exhibitions in 2011 and 2012 in conjunction with the 50th anniversary of the withdrawal of thalidomide from the market, which were held in several countries, including Germany, Britain, Australia, Ireland, Belgium, Netherlands, Austria, Spain and Italy, bore witness to the high levels of frustration and anger among groups of survivors and their families in particular.

Not surprisingly, more than five decades after the drug was withdrawn from sale in most markets around the world in the wake of overwhelming evidence that it was causing birth defects to thousands and killing thousands more in the womb, the thalidomide catastrophe still carries with it powerful emotional resonance along with a strong

[1] Medizinisch Pharmazeutische Studiengesellschaft e.V., Dokumentation III/71, 'Schriftlicher Einstellungsbeschluß der Ersten Großen Strafkammer des Landgerichts Aachen im sog. Contergan-Verfahren' (Frankfurt, 1971). For the point about the longest trial in German legal history, see p. 70.

desire among many to try to explain just what happened. Aspects of its unfolding and aftermath have therefore formed the focus of sustained medical and scientific inquiry, and the catastrophe has also stimulated careful historical scrutiny, impassioned personal testimony, heroic investigative journalism and numerous documentary films. Nevertheless, even after more than half a century of scrutiny and more than six decades since the start of the catastrophe, there are still a large number of mysterious circumstances surrounding its origins, how it developed and what happened in its aftermath. Questions remain, for instance, about such issues as:

- how and why a family firm focused on cosmetics and soaps decided to establish a pharmaceutical company, Chemie Grünenthal, in the context of Germany in the immediate aftermath of the Second World War;
- how that firm was able to afford not only the costs of the trial of its executives but also the settlement that was offered towards the end of it;
- and how it continued to market the drug even after the disaster.

But, perhaps more astonishingly, in spite of the sustained attention to thalidomide by scholars and the media over several decades, a comprehensive account of the drug – one that critically examines its origins, its makers and marketers, its victims, its withdrawal from widespread sale, the trial and the circumstances surrounding its suspension, the campaigns for justice that have continued after that and the drug's continued impact even after its 'withdrawal' – remains outstanding and is long overdue. This book is meant to examine some of these mysteries, often on the basis of sources that have never been used before, and it is also meant to provide, for the first time, a full account of the 'career' of this devastating drug.

Still, writing such a comprehensive account and trying to solve a range of lingering mysteries in the process were not our intention when we started the research that has resulted in this book. Instead, these emerged as our aims over time, as did the specific emphases and themes of the chapters that follow. How the team of authors was formed and how and why the focus of our research changed, sometimes substantially, are therefore central to understanding the story we tell and the way we tell it.

In 2007, Martin Johnson was director of the Thalidomide Trust, the UK charity set up to administer the compensation paid to thalidomide victims by the Distillers Company (later Diageo). In addition to his other duties, he was continuing to provide support for activists from the thalidomide community. After all, many thalidomiders, by that time well into their forties, had begun to suffer not only from their original injuries, but also from the long-term effects of having to deal with them. As they got older, this would only get worse, and therefore more expensive. At the same time, the funding available to support them was already proving inadequate, although campaigning by thalidomide activists led in 2005 to an agreement with Diageo to provide considerably more cash to the Trust, which was also guaranteed over a longer period of time. Still, the campaigners were not at all satisfied that justice had been done. Although UK thalidomiders were by 2006 beginning to receive payments that were more in keeping with their actual needs, those outside the UK were not. And, there was also considerable feeling among the activists that key organisations that had been involved in causing the disaster should be held to account. Attention therefore turned to campaigns directed at the UK government, and, even more centrally, at the firm at the heart of the devastation, Chemie Grünenthal. By the end of January 2008, the new targets of the campaign led to the formation of the International Contergan Thalidomide Alliance (ICTA), an activist movement uniting a wide range of UK and European survivors of the drug (Contergan was Grünenthal's trade name for thalidomide in Germany and in some other markets).

In the meantime, Chemie Grünenthal was coming under pressure not just from activists, but also from the media, most importantly in the form of a docu-drama about the thalidomide disaster, 'Eine einzige Tablette' ('Just a single tablet'), which aired on German television in November 2007 and which painted the firm in a very bad light. The film also had an effect on the eventual writing of this book: it spurred a second co-author, Tobias Arndt, to take up contact with thalidomide campaigners, offering his services to them, something which initially involved using his considerable skills in researching and interpreting patents and later the deployment of skill and perseverance in ferreting out crucial historical documents in the archives.

Collecting, collating and analysing the various thalidomide patents served as the catalyst for the next crucial stage in the genesis of this book. When some of the findings were presented at a meeting of the Thalidomide Trust in Leeds in October 2008, the Trust's Medical Adviser, Dr. C.G.H. Newman, asked an apparently straightforward question that does not seem to have occurred to anyone previously:

> *How did the authors of the patent specification know the detailed information about the effects of the drug on humans?*

The question – how did they know? – took on particular significance given the fact that the analysis of the original patent from 1954 also revealed that it was registered very shortly after the drug was allegedly first discovered, in other words *before any extensive testing to determine the drug's effects could possibly have been carried out.*

Trying to answer that question formed the first item on the research agenda that has led in the end to this book. The only possible way to do so was to look backward, and, of course, one does not have to look too far backward from 1954 in German history to find instances of extensive testing of drugs, often on human subjects, and often against their will or without their knowledge. The suspicion that there might be something to the idea that the detailed information on the effects of thalidomide on humans in the patent had come from testing on human subjects that had been carried out during the National Socialist period soon appeared to be borne out by a number of startling facts. One of them revolved around the chief scientist of Chemie Grünenthal, Dr. Heinrich Mückter, who had been working for much of the war at the Army Institute for Typhus and Virus Research in Kraków, a research institute which tested various drugs on inmates at the Buchenwald concentration camp. The second involved the discovery of documents linking the much more prominent, although also shadowy, figure of Otto Ambros directly to Chemie Grünenthal, although the nature of that relationship and its connection to thalidomide was not entirely clear. During the Nazi period, Ambros had been a high-ranking member of the managing board of IG Farbenindustrie AG, a massive chemical firm that not only supplied the Nazi war machine with crucial goods such as synthetic oil and rubber, but also, notoriously, built an integrated chemical production facility near the death camp at Auschwitz using slave labour. Ambros, in fact, was the board member primarily responsible for the IG Auschwitz project, and he was duly found guilty in the IG Farben Nuremberg Trial in 1948. He was sentenced to eight years in prison for his crimes. Changing priorities in the occupation of Germany, however, mainly owing to the Cold War, led to a change in attitude toward some war criminals, and Ambros was released from prison after just three years by order of American High Commissioner John McCloy. Although Ambros agreed not to serve on the boards of any of the large successors to IG Farben (which included the company he had started working for during the 1920s, BASF, as well as Bayer and Hoechst), his status as a war criminal clearly did not impede his return to prominence in the German and international business communities. Already during the 1950s, he not only served as a highly paid consultant for firms abroad such as W.R. Grace in the United States and the Distillers Company in Britain, he also served on the boards of a number of German firms, such as pharmaceutical producer Knoll AG, where Herman Wirtz was a board member, and eventually (although much later), Grünenthal itself.

These and other discoveries led Martin Johnson to seek additional expertise in the area of German industrial and business history, and he turned to Professor Richard Evans, at that time Regius Professor of History at Cambridge University, for advice. Evans suggested that Johnson contact Professor Raymond G. Stokes at the Centre for Business History in Scotland at the University of Glasgow because he had worked extensively on the history of IG Farben for a number of years. He became the final member of the team of authors in 2009.

Although we should state clearly at the outset that we have found no proof whatsoever in the course of our research since 2008 that thalidomide originated in the Nazi period, our investigation into the drug's 'Nazi connections' has nevertheless proved fruitful. For one thing, we have been able to highlight the centrality of Werner Schulemann, Professor of Pharmacology and Toxicology at the University of Bonn, in the unfolding of the thalidomide story, a role that began during the Nazi period and continued well into the post-war period. More importantly, though, we have been able to reconstruct networks of individuals and organisations as well as the emergence of patterns of behaviour established during the Nazi period which continued into the post-war period and had a major impact on the origins and unfolding of the thalidomide catastrophe. These findings are presented in Chapter 2.

What became clear as we thought more deeply about these findings, though, was that the roots of the thalidomide catastrophe in the Nazi period – although extremely important – did not constitute the main issue here. As suggested in the preceding paragraph, it was a combination of continuities, but also some major changes in the post-war period, which led to the catastrophe. In other words, we realised that this was *not* primarily a story about 'the last Nazi war crime', but rather one that centred not only on astonishing levels of corporate irresponsibility, cover-up, collusion and corruption, but also on the quest for justice by survivors and their families, all of this over a very long period of time. The main focus of research and thinking, then, turned to the years from the early 1950s to the present, and we also began to think in terms of a book covering the entire history of the drug and its impact, from National Socialism to the most recent past.

A number of additional factors contributed to this recalibration. For one thing, better scientific understanding of the mechanisms through which thalidomide affects the human body, and in particular the foetus, along with better data about the international dimensions of the catastrophe, meant that we have been able, for the first time, to produce estimates of its true extent and of the ways in which earlier withdrawal of the drug would have reduced the number of victims. This, together with testimony from survivors, their families and others involved in the disaster as it unfolded, allows us to provide an overview of both what has been and what might have been in this very 'preventable disaster', which forms the subject of Chapter 1. We then go on in Chapters 3-5 to investigate other aspects of the emergence of the catastrophe in the post-war period, focusing on the establishment of Chemie Grünenthal (Ch.3), the discovery of thalidomide (Ch.4) and the cover-up and conspiracy involved in attempting to evade the eventual withdrawal of the drug from sale in late 1961 (Ch.5).

The other factors affecting the change in emphasis in our research involved two interrelated developments. On the one hand, we have been influenced by our connections with the activists involved in trying to achieve justice for thalidomide survivors around the world as they have sought to hold not just governments, but also companies – and in particular Chemie Grünenthal – to full account for this tragedy. On the other hand, the activists' interests have helped lead to, but also been in turn shaped by, our discovery of a range of primary documents that have never been used before in relation to the history of thalidomide.

Here, the records of the prosecution in the trial that took place in Germany between 1968 and 1970, which include a large amount of material that was collected but never presented at the trial, have been extremely valuable. More recently, attention to the role of the German federal government in bringing the trial to an end has led to the discovery of important documents in Germany's national and state archives. The story of the trial and its suspension is examined critically on the basis of this important new evidence in Chapter 6.

The trial did not result in justice in any meaningful way, in spite of the creation soon after its suspension of a foundation in Germany to compensate victims. Chapter 7 uses a range of new sources to examine alternative paths taken to try to achieve justice, not just in Germany, but in several different countries, as well as the outcomes of those attempts. Chapter 8 deals with what happened to thalidomide after the 'withdrawal' of the drug in 1961. As we show, Chemie Grünenthal and its licensees never actually stopped selling it, with the result, among other things, that thalidomide continues to damage children in many parts of the Third World. Brazil, for instance, experienced a new wave of thalidomide births in the 1970s, with the most recent child affected being born in 2010. The final chapter presents some conclusions on the basis of this extraordinary story, which has many extremely depressing, frustrating and anger-inducing elements to it, but which is also sometimes surprisingly uplifting.

Figure 1: Ed, aged 3, at the garage where his father worked as a bus driver.

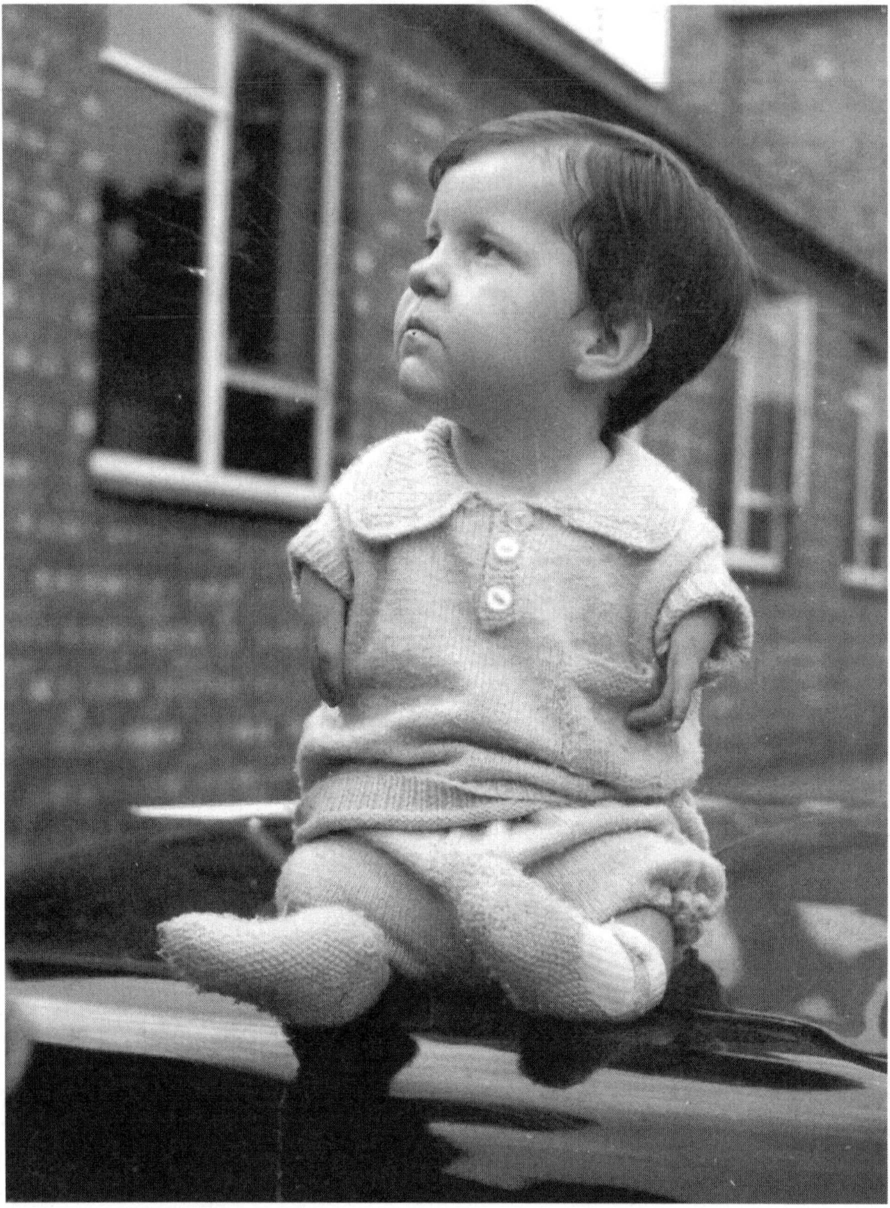

Chapter One

A Preventable Disaster

How the entire disaster could have been prevented and more than 100,00 babies saved.

WHEN PEOPLE CONSIDER THE WORLD'S worst man-made peace-time disasters, the 2,996 deaths that resulted directly from the 9/11 attacks on New York City will spring to the mind of many, while others will think of the sinking of the *Titanic* in 1912, when 1,514 lost their lives. Others still might suggest the gas leak at the Bhopal plant of Union Carbide in 1984, which caused the deaths of perhaps 11,000 inhabitants in the surrounding area. Other candidates might include disasters where the numbers affected are less certain, such as the case of the anti-arthritis drug Vioxx, which very probably caused several thousand people to die prematurely of strokes and heart attacks between 1999 and 2004. Or there is the case of the asbestos industry, which probably inflicted the greatest toll of premature deaths around the world in this entire catalogue of disasters over the course of about a century: in the United Kingdom alone, an estimated 4,700 people lost their lives owing to asbestos through 2011.[2] Many more died from the effects of asbestos elsewhere around the world.

In terms of direct loss of life and long-term devastation, however, the thalidomide disaster exceeds all of these events, with the exception of the case of asbestos. But given that thalidomide wreaked most of its havoc over the space of just five years, the drug's trail of death and destruction was more concentrated than even that of asbestos. Moreover, the thalidomide disaster not only exceeds most of these other

2 *http://www.hse.gov.uk/statistics/causdis/asbestos.htm* <accessed 2 July 2014>.

events in the total number of deaths, but also in the terrible injuries inflicted on surviving children, the impact on their families and the long-term consequences of these initial injuries. Then, too, a less well-known form of devastation resulting from the drug involved a large number of adult victims who experienced severe and long-term nerve damage.

In this chapter, we start by estimating the total number of deaths caused by the drug. We then go on to explain how large numbers of victims – both those who died and those who survived – could have been spared, even very late in the day, had Chemie Grünenthal, the company that manufactured, sold and licensed the drug, acted on the many warnings its managers received. Finally, we detail the effects of the disaster on survivors, their families and on society more generally, many of which persist into the present day.

Counting the victims

Between 1958 and 1962, tens of thousands of women throughout the world endured the devastating experience of finding that the baby they were carrying unaccountably miscarried, or, perhaps even worse, of being told after they gave birth that their baby was stillborn. Moreover, many of the mothers of stillborn babies never learned of the severe deformities their dead children had because it was not customary in those days to show them to the mother. The difficulty in uncovering the full death toll caused by thalidomide, then, begins with the unrecorded numbers of miscarriages and stillbirths, and the practice of infanticide, which was commonplace at the time.

But there are ways of estimating the number of deaths, indeed on the basis of survivors. As we know, thousands of other mothers discovered that the baby they had so eagerly anticipated had severe birth defects, sometimes with missing or severe reductions to arms and/or legs, or even worse, damage to their internal organs, including hearts, kidneys, intestines, genitals etc. Moreover, this problem did not afflict a narrow section of any society. In Britain, for instance, the women who gave birth to a thalidomide baby ranged from a dockside prostitute to a viscountess. A similar range of women was affected elsewhere, too. Some of them never got over the shock of this experience; all found their lives and expectations changed irrevocably.

Early in 1962, following the withdrawal of the drug in November 1961 in most countries where its use had previously been approved, counting began of the living children born damaged by the drug. A number of estimates were subsequently put forward, but the only verified and complete counts are those compiled by and for the national compensation schemes established in the 1970s in Germany, Britain, Japan, Sweden, Australia and, much later, Brazil. In other words, we only know for certain about the numbers of those who survived long enough to be deemed eligible, by experts appointed for this purpose, to participate in national compensation schemes. We know nothing about the exact numbers of those victims who died before that, nor about those who may have been affected by the drug, but were deemed ineligible to participate. Finally, we know very little about the numbers of survivors in those countries such as Spain where the drug was used but where no national compensation scheme was put in place until 2010, and where only a handful of survivors has so far qualified for support.

Still, the verified numbers of survivors in selected countries can serve as a basis for estimates for total numbers affected by using a variety of supporting evidence.

COUNTING SURVIVORS

The number of survivors who were damaged by versions of the drug supplied directly by Chemie Grünenthal in West Germany, the Netherlands, Austria, Ireland, Belgium and Finland and registered by the German Contergan Trust was 2,901 by December 2011. In other countries that eventually implemented compensation schemes, the drug was manufactured and supplied under licence. For the UK, for instance, where thalidomide was produced under licence by the Distillers Company[3], the official total number of survivors by December 2011 was 524. In Japan, there were 309, in Scandinavia 133 and in Canada 104. 45 were registered in Australia before 2010, and reportedly a further 105 have since been accepted. In Brazil, where a second wave of thalidomide birth defects began in the 1970s, more than 600 have been

3 A report from Grünenthal dated March 1960 coupled with a meeting minute from 6 February 1964 indicate that Grünenthal probably supplied most if not all the bulk thalidomide which Distillers made into pills, syrups and suppositories for their customers. Landesarchiv Nordrheinwestfalen – Abteilung Rheinland (LAV NRW R) Duisberg – Gerichte Rep. 139 Nr. 26 Bl. 207; LAV NRW R, Gerichte Rep. 139 Nr. 60 Bl. 022-028.

registered by the government, with thalidomide births recorded there as recently as 2010. People working to support the Brazilian survivors say that there are a large number of non-registered cases, and that the real total is around 1,000.[4]

But there were victims – and survivors – in other countries where national compensation schemes do not exist or have come into existence only recently, and even in places such as the United States, where the drug was never approved for sale by the Food and Drug Administration (FDA). It was only in October 2007, for instance, that the Spanish government admitted that thalidomide had been available in Spain into at least the mid-1960s. A year later, in October 2008, the Italian government announced a scheme to compensate thalidomide victims in the country. While the full numbers for Spain and Italy remain uncertain, a combined total of about 370 people had been registered as thalidomiders in the two countries through early 2012, with estimates of total survivors in each case amounting to 500. A substantial but unknown number of survivors are located in Central America (probably over 100), while in the USA itself some 40 survivors are believed to have made successful claims for compensation.[5]

To arrive at estimates of the full extent of the damage in countries such as Italy and Spain, it is useful to note that distribution of the drug there covered much the same period as in the UK, Sweden and Ireland, i.e. just under four years in total starting in 1958.[6] The UK, with a population in 1960 of approximately 50 million, had some 500 registered survivors as of 2011, while Sweden, with approximately 9 million inhabitants, had nearly 100 survivors. For its part, Ireland, with 3.5 million citizens in 1960, had 35 survivors. If those remarkably

4 Figures collated by the Thalidomide Trust 2001-2013 from a variety of sources, including reports from the Conterganstiftung, Ishizue Foundation, Foreningen fur die Nevrosedynskadade, Taionlus, TVAC.

5 This number was an estimate provided by Thalidomide Victim's Association of Canada based on their contacts in the USA. Dr. C.G.H. Newman writes: 'Dick (Prof. R. W.) Smithells passed an invitation to me to go to the USA and take part as an expert witness in a battle between Merrel Dow [known as Richardson Merrell until 1980] (for the defense) and a Mr Traci, an attorney who had won 20 or more claims for compensation. The index claim in which I became involved, and as far as I can recall all the others of whom I got details had malformations quite unlike thalidomide embryopathy, and eventually the judge agreed. The number of actual USA thalidomiders is therefore likely to be much smaller.' Private email to author Martin Johnson, 13 December 2016.

6 The drug was officially withdrawn in most of these countries in November 1961, although there are claims that it was available in Spain into the 1980s. See James Badcock, 'Spain's forgotten Thalidomide victims see glimmer of hope', *BBC News,* 23 December 2016: *http://www.bbc.co.uk/news/world-38386021* <12 June 2017>.

consistent ratios apply to Italy and Spain as well, the combined total for those two countries could therefore be as high as 1,000. The combination of recorded figures and best estimates indicates that the total number of thalidomiders surviving beyond childhood around the world is in the range of about 6,000, as detailed in Table 1.1.

Table 1.1: Thalidomide survivors beyond childhood worldwide (registered survivors and estimates as compiled in 2003).

Country	Verified numbers of survivors	Estimated number of survivors
Chemie Grünenthal direct supplies (Germany and five other countries)	2,901	
UK	524	
Japan	309	
Scandinavia	133	
Canada	104	
Australia	150	
Brazil	600+	1,000
Italy	350	500
Spain	23	500
US		40+
Latin America ex-Brazil		100+
Total	**5024+**	**6261+***

Source: Figures collated by the Thalidomide Trust 2001-2013 from a variety of sources, including reports from the Conterganstiftung, Ishizue Foundation, Foreningen fur die Nevrosedynskadade, Taionlus, TVAC.

* *This figure is the total of estimated plus verified survivors in the countries listed.*

But again, it is important to underscore that these figures represent those who survived long enough to be registered under compensation schemes (or, in some cases, estimates of those who would have been registered). We do not know for sure how many thalidomide-affected children were born, but anecdotal and other evidence suggest the numbers were much larger.

An important example indicating the potential scale of this undercounting took place at the funeral of Julie Merritt in Treorchy, South Wales, in January 2006. The elderly minister conducting the service commented afterwards that he had known Julie all her life, going on to comment that, 'She must have been the last Thalidomide baby from the Rhondda.' He continued, 'I remember there were at least thirty of them.'[7] But the UK records show only two Thalidomide Trust beneficiaries born in the Rhondda Valley area – and the other one had moved away. In any event, the undercounting of babies who were not counted officially as thalidomiders includes those who died shortly after childbirth from their injuries or from what was essentially infanticide, those who died within the first year of birth and those who did not live long enough to be registered under compensation schemes.

Let us start with those who died shortly after birth. Kim Morton, a prominent British thalidomider, was contacted after a public event by a woman who asked how Kim's legs were when she was born, and was told they were bent up behind her back. The woman burst into tears, and she said her baby had legs like that, as they had been described to her. She had given birth, and the baby was taken away from her; she wasn't allowed to see it. 'They told me he was stillborn – but I heard him cry,' she said. She asked for a post-mortem examination, but the doctor told her that her son's body had been destroyed in her own kitchen fire.[8]

Some others were left to die of exposure, while others still were suffocated. One doctor recalled seeing the midwife, out of sight of the mother, push a four-limb damaged baby, who was in a small box and not breathing, underneath the delivery bed. The doctor inadvertently kicked the box with his foot, and the baby started crying and survives to this day. The shame of being party to this stayed with that doctor until his dying days. The baby in the box was Kevin Donnellon, who went on to achieve an education to postgraduate level, become a university lecturer, a campaigner against cruise missiles and a father.[9]

Claudia Schmidt-Herterich, a German Contergan survivor, tells of meeting a doctor in the mid-1980s:

[7] Conversation between Reverend Cyril Llewellyn and Martin Johnson on 20 January 2006.

[8] Kim Morton, Beatrice Atcheson, *Kim – A True Story* (Londonderry: Causeway press, 1996) pp. 153-156.

[9] Confidential conversation with the doctor concerned reported by A. Summerside, Development Director of Thalidomide Trust, April 2002.

In 1984 I took part in a meeting of the CDU Federal Committee on Social Policy as the administrative advisor for German disabled students. During the break in that meeting a man in his sixties came to me and asked me if I was a thalidomider. Of course, I said yes! He asked me if I would talk outside of the room with him. I agreed and went out with him where he told me that he used to be a doctor in charge in a hospital in North Rhine Westphalia. He saw a lot of babies born with deformed limbs in 1960, 1961 and 1962. He explained how horrified the doctors and the staff were trying to help those deformed babies to live. And now he started crying! He then said that at this hospital the severely deformed babies mostly did not survive, because they left them lying starving because they were sure that we would not be able to live. They told the parents that the baby was born dead!

Now, having met me, he knew, he had done wrong... And he kept on telling me that there were other directors of different hospitals he knew who did the same! I do not need to tell you how awful I felt, knowing that so many babies could have lived even though they were 'deformed' like me! [10]

In Belgium, there is a well documented case of infanticide of a thalidomide baby. Suzanne van der Put, who gave birth to a baby girl in May 1962 with no arms and the anal canal emptying through her vagina, killed her newborn with an overdose of barbiturates when her daughter was just one week old. She was put on trial for murder, but in November 1962 was found not guilty, even though the fact that she had deliberately killed the baby was not disputed. 500 spectators in the courtroom cheered the verdict, and a public opinion poll ran 10 to 1 in favour of the mother's acquittal.[11]

But even those thalidomide babies who were born and not put to death often did not survive for long. Neonatal mortality rates were high. Jane McKinnon was one of the victims. Born on 15 March 1961, Jane lived for just four days, dying in her mother's arms because of a heart defect. Fifty years later, her mother (who was never able to have

10 Email from Claudia Schmidt-Herterich to Martin Johnson, 2 December 2011, 18:50.

11 'Medicine: Thalidomide homicide', *Time* (16 November 1962), available at: *http://www.time.com/time/magazine/article/0,9171,829419,00.html* <viewed 10 November 2014>.

another child) said that she had thought of her baby 'with such a beautiful face' every day since.[12] Elizabeth Grant, her parents' first child, was born in January 1960, but lived for only six days and died of intestinal atresia, which meant that her intestines were blocked, and potentially very underdeveloped beyond the blockage. Fifty years later, her father wrote how he believed that even though he and his wife had gone on to have three healthy children, the loss of this first baby had contributed to his wife's poor mental health decades later in the years before she passed away.[13]

The German expert Professor Widukind Lenz, who played a key role in the identification and documentation of the thalidomide disaster, and his British counterpart, Professor Richard W. Smithells, separately estimated that between 40% and 45% of all the thalidomide babies born alive died before their first birthdays.[14] Of one group of 31 thalidomide babies born with intestinal atresia, only 12 were still alive in 1964. Congenital heart deformities were also common, but again, few survived: only 19 out of 45 reported with this problem were still alive by 1964.[15] In other words, the estimates of survivors provided in Table 1.1 need to be revised sharply upward to include all children born alive with thalidomide damage.

But there are reasons for increasing the estimates of these numbers still further. After all, many who survived for a longer period following their birth died before they could be registered for the settlement schemes. As Leigh Gath, a thalidomider from Northern Ireland recalled:

> *12 [thalidomide] babies were apparently born at Daisy Hill Hospital, Newry, between 1960-62. I think I was the last. One of the kids was called Anne McKevitt. Two others I know of were called Flood and McComiskey. The Flood baby died aged 1 or 2, the McComiskey baby died in infancy. Davy Thompson died when he was about 7-8.*[16]

However, although we know that Anne McKevitt died aged 14 in 1975, children by the names of Flood, McComiskey and David

12 Telephone call from mother to Martin Johnson, January 2010.

13 Letter from father, Dr. Robert L. Grant, to Martin Johnson, January 2010.

14 W. Lenz, 'A Short History of Thalidomide Teratology', *Teratology* 38:203-215 (1988); R.W. Smithells, C.G.H. Newman, 'Recognition of Thalidomide Defects', *J. Med. Gen.* 1992; 29; 716-723.

15 Ministry of Health, *Reports on Public Health and Medical Subjects No. 112: Deformities Caused by Thalidomide* (London: Her Majesty's Stationery Office, 1964) pp. 46, 48.

16 Email from Leigh Gath to Martin Johnson, 13 June 2008, 16:07.

Thompson were never registered by the Thalidomide Trust, and must therefore have died before 1973. All in all, this meant that three out of the twelve thalidomide babies born alive in one hospital were not registered because they did not live long enough, a ratio of 1 in 4. On the other hand, one Ministry of Health report shows the early death toll was even higher: out of one group of 201 thalidomide children born between 1960 and 1962, 70 had already died by 1964, i.e. a ratio of more than 1 in 3.[17] A London-based paediatric expert confirms this, estimating that about one third of the thalidomide children he had treated did not reach their teenage years.[18]

Although we have a substantial amount of anecdotal evidence and informed estimates, arriving at an overall approximation of the number of babies affected by thalidomide who were born alive is difficult. But we can start with an overall estimate of 2,000 thalidomide babies born in the UK that Professor Smithells, one of the key British figures in the identification and documentation of the thalidomide disaster, came up with by taking into consideration his best estimates of those who died within their first year, those who died before the compensation scheme plus those who entered the compensation scheme.[19] In other words, three-quarters of these survivors must have died before their teens because the total number registered by the Thalidomide Trust in Britain from 1973 until 2011 was only 524. If we assume that this rate of attrition held for other countries as well, we can come up with an overall estimate of live births of children affected by thalidomide by taking the figures in Table 1.1 and multiplying them by four. Table 1.2 provides an overview of these estimates by country.

HOW MANY MISCARRIAGES AND STILLBIRTHS?

On the basis of these statistics on survivors, we can begin to estimate the numbers of children who died *before they were born* as a result of thalidomide, i.e. babies whose mothers miscarried or were stillborn because of the drug. We use two different methods for doing that.

[17] Ministry of Health, *Deformities Caused by Thalidomide,* pp. 46, 48.
[18] Private conversation Dr. C.G.H. Newman with Martin Johnson, circa 2010.
[19] Conversation Professor Smithells with Martin Johnson, November 2001.

Table 1.2: Estimated total number of children born alive who were affected by thalidomide.

Country	Estimated number of live births
Chemie Grünenthal direct supplies (Germany and five other countries)	11,604
UK	2,096
Japan	1,236
Scandinavia	532
Canada	416
Australia	600
Brazil	4,000
Italy	2,000
Spain	2,000
US	160+
Latin America ex-Brazil	400+
Total	**25,044+**

Source: Calculated on the basis of figures in Table 1.1 for registrants in national compensation schemes and estimated longer-term survivals in other countries/regions.

A 1952 experiment with a drug named Aminopterin, which also causes serious birth defects and has some chemical similarities to thalidomide, produced 10 stillbirths/miscarriages out of the 12 pregnant women who were given it, a survival ratio of 2 out of 12, or 1 in 6.[20] Because of the close similarities between Aminopterin and one of the primary break-down products (metabolites) of thalidomide, it is reasonable to expect that thalidomide could have had similar effects. And, if this survival ratio is applied to the totals for thalidomide live births in Table 1.2 above, the estimated number of babies who did not

[20] J.B. Thiersch, F.S. Philips (1950) 'Effect of 4-amino-pteroylglutamic acid (aminopterin) on early pregnancy', *Proceedings of the Society for Experimental Biology and Medicine,* 1950, May, 74(1): pp. 204-208.

survive to live birth amounted to more than 150,264, with the total number of babies affected (including all who were born alive) upwards of 175,000. Moreover, the dosage rate of Aminopterin in this trial was barely a quarter of the normal minimum dose of thalidomide (5-6 milligrams [mg], against the normal tablet size for thalidomide of 25-100 mg). Thus, the figures for thalidomide are likely to be conservative, and could easily be doubled.

Other evidence suggests that those babies born alive probably represent between 10% and 40% of those exposed to thalidomide in the womb, with the remainder being miscarried or stillborn.[21] In other words, using this technique for estimating the total number of babies who did not survive birth could range from 62,600 (if those born alive represented 40% of all those exposed to thalidomide in the womb) to over 250,000 (if those born alive represented 10%), with total number affected (including survivors) ranging from 87,600 to about 275,500.

Even the minimum estimates presented here represent a very large number of babies affected in a very short time, and it should be emphasized that even the maximum estimate presented here is likely to be conservative. And these figures in turn represent individual cases of pain and suffering that affected not just the babies concerned, but also families. Just to illustrate the human experience behind the numbers, let us take a look at one example among the wide range of qualitative evidence on stillbirth of thalidomide babies. As Patrick Pope, a UK thalidomider, said in 2003:

> *I was one of twins, you know. My twin was stillborn. The nurses told my mother he was 'flushed away'. They told my mother there were four other thalidomide babies stillborn in that hospital on the same day.*[22]

The nurses who spoke to Patrick's mother, of course, could not have known that thalidomide was to blame, but it is important in terms of context that they were experiencing a considerable number of stillbirths

21 Müller, W. (1969) 'Slaughter of the Innocent', *Münchner Medizinische Wochenschrift,* No. 34, repr. in Ruesch, H., *Slaughter of the Innocent* (Civitas, 1983) p. 365. Early mortality rates are also evidenced in: 'Public Health – Congenital Abnormalities due to Thalidomide'; *The Lancet* (3 November 1962) p. 931; and Dawkins, M. (letter), 'Thalidomide and Congenital Abnormalities', *The Lancet* (9 March 1963) pp. 552-553.

22 Conversation with Patrick Pope during visit by Martin Johnson, 8 September 2003. Patrick Pope's painful and harrowing early life was reported: *The Sunday Times* Insight Team, *Suffer The Children: The Story of Thalidomide* (New York: Viking Press, 1979) pps. 118, 183, 214-215.

of babies who were clearly deformed or damaged. Moreover, Patrick's mother was also told it was normal for such babies to be 'turned over' (i.e. left to die). There was no general system for recording stillborn deformed babies at the time,[23] but in Liverpool, where Professor Smithells started a register of congenital abnormalities, records of thirty cases of limb-deficient babies from the thalidomide period showed that eleven were stillborn or died soon after birth.[24] This evidence simply confirms yet again that large numbers of thalidomide babies were stillborn.

The injuries inflicted

The records of British, German and Swedish national thalidomide compensation organisations show that between establishment (1971-75) and 2010, approximately 10% of registered thalidomide survivors died. This is more than double the death rate expected for a UK equivalent population of the same age group over that period.[25] It is not surprising, though, in light of the damage suffered by the survivors.

The most severely damaged survivors have four-limb damage, and are blind with various forms of brain damage. This was the almost inevitable result if a mother took a tablet each day from around the 20th to the 30th day after conception. A tablet on days 21-22 could result in loss of, or damage to, the eyes. For days 22-23, intake of thalidomide could result in similar damage to the ears and face, whereas one tablet on day 24 could result in a complete absence of arms, and on day 29 an absence of legs. It is likely that the most severely damaged survivors were a tiny fraction of those living through such trauma; the majority damaged to this degree could not have survived.

A diagram of the range of limb damage was worked out on the basis of X-rays by the German experts Professors H.-L. Henkel and H.-G. Willert.[26] (See Figure 2.) This shows typical leg and arm damage, beginning on the left with the lowest level of damage, with the greatest level on the far right. It is clear from the diagram that as the damage

23 Ministry of Health, *Deformities Caused by Thalidomide,* pp. 4, 5, 11.

24 *Ibid.,* p. 5.

25 From mortality data held by the Thalidomide Trust (UK), the Conterganstiftung (Germany) and the Föreningen fur de Nevrosedinskadade (Sweden) compared against the British Actuarial table, 'English Life Table 14'.

26 H.-L. Henkel, H.-G. Willert (1968) 'Dysmelia; a Classification and a Pattern in a Group of Congenital Malformations of the Limbs', *Journal of Bone and Joint Surgery,* August 1969, pp. 399-414.

progresses, it affects every bone in the upper limb system from the shoulder blade to the finger, and in the lower limb system from the pelvis to the toes. The arm only has to be slightly reduced for the shoulder joint to disappear completely, which means that the experience of the survivor is likely to be of living with a shoulder that dislocates easily, or may be permanently dislocated. The experience of the survivor with relatively slight leg damage may be that when the use of his or her hip has become unbearably painful, s/he will be told that there is not enough bone structure to fix an artificial hip joint to, or that the pelvic girdle is not actually 'joined up' as a normal rigid structure, but instead held together by flexible cartilage. Although not so obvious from the diagram, there is a tendency with leg-system damage for the number of toes to increase, while the number of fingers is reduced. This is encapsulated in the title of the autobiography of Rosie Moriarty-Simmonds, a survivor who has no arms, hands or legs, but still has 'four fingers and thirteen toes'.[27]

Figure 2: Teratological sequence of dysmelia of the upper and lower extremities.

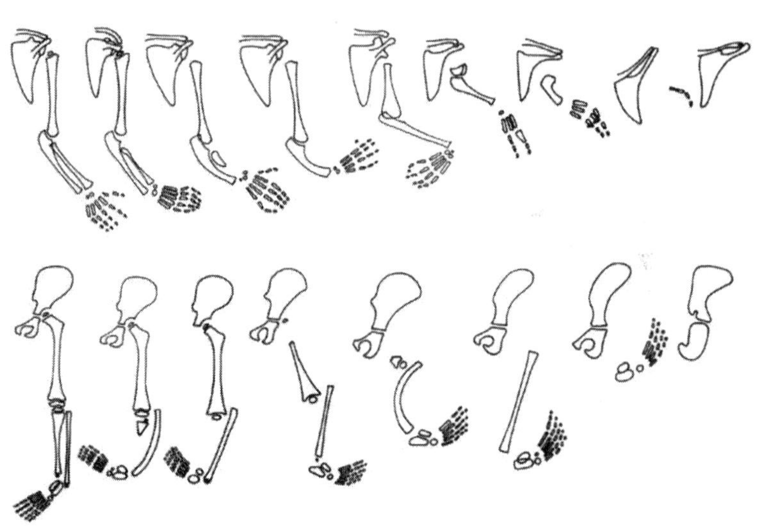

Source: H.-L. Henkel, H.-G. Willert (1968), 'Dysmelia; a Classification and a Pattern in a Group of Congenital Malformations of the Limbs', Journal of Bone and Joint Surgery, August 1969, pp. 399-414.

27 Rosaleen Moriarty-Simmonds, *Four Fingers and Thirteen Toes* (Cardiff: R. Moriarty Simmonds, 2007), ISBN 09548883-2-4.

This teratological sequence did not just affect foetal development; it often went on to affect the everyday life of the victim. Julie Lane, for instance, was born with a full set of limbs, and minor hand damage. But her disabilities were extensive nevertheless. For one thing, she suffered severe damage to her ears, and therefore relied on powerful hearing aids before losing her hearing altogether in the last four or five years of her life, which ended at age 44. Moreover, from an early age she started having epileptic-type fits. She then lost the use of her legs in her early teens, and used a wheelchair from that point forward. She did her best to enjoy her life to the full, but the fits got worse as she got older. Unfortunately, because electroencephalograph (EEG) tests did not show the patterns of brain activity typical of epilepsy, her mother reported that an unnamed consultant neurologist had confidently said that her fits were psychosomatic. This stigmatised Julie ('it's all in her mind, poor thing...') and led to an uphill battle for her and her family to get the proper nursing care she needed. As she turned forty, she started losing the strength in her arms, and her already poor eyesight deteriorated rapidly. In her final year, she estimated that without medication she would have been experiencing 20-30 fits a day. What was worse was that by then she could only communicate by lip reading, at which she had become very skilful, except she knew she was now going blind.[28] She died aged just 44. The post-mortem examination of her brain showed evidence of major internal damage, which had been there from before birth – thalidomide destroyed her practically from the 'inside out' via her nervous system.

Dominic Galvin is another survivor with a similar level of damage to Julie Lane, except his eyesight and hearing were largely unimpaired. The central brain damage for him, though, has had the effect of making his speech very difficult, and his control over his limbs has always been poor. The result is that strangers treat him as if he has a severe learning disability, which for someone whose IQ was measured at 138 when he was a child is very difficult to bear. Damage to his oesophagus (gullet) and trachea (windpipe) has meant that his feeding must be done with great care because otherwise food would end up in his lungs and kill him. His mother Sadie, a qualified nurse, provided him with 24-hour

[28] Thalidomide Trust Visit Reports ref 203 dated 23.11.2000; 20.06.2001; 27.03.2006. Julie Lane's mother Pat fought hard to get adequate support for Julie all her life. Some of that battle involved tackling Enoch Powell (to no effect!). It is reported in: *The Sunday Times* Insight Team, *Suffer The Children: The Story of Thalidomide,* pp. 137-141.

care for over 55 years until her death in March 2015.[29] He is now cared for by another relative.

Those survivors whose damage is mainly to their nervous systems or other internal organs find that others do not recognise the severity of their damage. And yet, thalidomide frequently caused anal atresia, which means the baby was born with a very restricted or absent anus. (Atresia, a word that appears frequently in descriptions of thalidomide damage, means simply that an organ is missing or that a bodily passage or orifice is completely blocked.) Emergency plastic surgery could correct these conditions in many cases and permit the survival of many of these babies (death took place in 7 days or fewer if this was not done), but the price of survival has often been lifelong incontinence of bowels, in other words a lifetime in nappies (diapers). When this is coupled to arms that are only 10-15 cm long, as is frequently the case, then 'cleaning yourself' becomes very difficult, if not impossible, unless you possess a 'paperless' toilet or have learned to use special portable implements.

In addition, a number of the girls discovered when they became women that their uterus was badly deformed or missing, with the consequent impact on hopes of having children. For some girls the anus and vagina joined a common orifice, and for a few there was no vagina at all ('vaginal atresia'). Some boys had corresponding degrees of damage to their genitals (e.g. Microphallus). These disabilities, with the most profound effects on how people live their lives, are not evident to strangers, but the mental suffering associated with them can be more severe than with much of the limb and other damage. There are other types of disability caused by thalidomide as well. For example, facial paralysis, partial or complete, is one effect of the drug, and is usually connected with eye and/or ear damage. Complete facial paralysis produces major social problems: 'We never know what he's thinking, what he wants or whether he likes something.'[30]

One effect of the disaster has been to extend the medical lexicon. The word 'phocomelia' was coined to describe thalidomide's signature effect of causing very short limbs and hands with no thumbs, looking like flippers: phocomelia literally (and bizarrely) means 'seal limb'. 'Amelia' means a complete absence of a limb, while another new word,

29 Thalidomide Trust Visit Reports ref. 137 dated 11.12.2002; 05.09.2007.

30 Parents of K., Thalidomide Trust beneficiary, full facial paralysis, brain damage and without speech, Thalidomide Trust Visit Reports ref. 279 dated 21.09.2000; 17.01.2001.

'dysmelia', was coined as a catch-all for any type of limb-reduction deformity. The medical lexicon already had a word 'dysmorphogenic' to describe something causing abnormal tissue growth (literal translation: different shape-causing), but the neologisms 'teratogen' and 'teratogenic' instead came into widespread use as a result of thalidomide, literally implying that drugs such as thalidomide were 'monster-making'. It seems as if some medical authorities viewed these disabled children as monsters.

Before we move on to consider the impact of this death and devastation on the families of the children involved, we should emphasize that there are also likely to be many who do not even suspect that their injuries were caused by thalidomide. After all, the drug was contained in medicines sold under a bewildering number of brand names (at least 49 different ones are known) and across a wide geographic span, including 19 European countries and at least 60 other countries worldwide.[31] What is more, in addition to birth defects, miscarriages, stillbirths and the deaths of infants and children that were caused by thalidomide, whether recorded or not recorded, a large number of adults suffered the nerve damage known as polyneuritis which was caused by the drug.[32] These injuries can be incapacitating and excruciatingly painful and are usually irreversible. In Germany by 1962, some 40,000 adults had been reported as affected. As many as 700,000 Germans were estimated to have taken the drug on a regular basis, and that makes it probable than a million or more in Europe as a whole may have done so. Given recent findings that between 20% and 70% of people taking it will develop peripheral neuropathy, the real

[31] Thalidomide distribution and births data collated with the aid of the Thalidomide Society (UK); from information received from the Thalidomide Victim's Association of Canada; the DLA Piper survey report for the Conterganstiftung, January 2012; from records of thalidomide distribution held by Chemie Grunenthal, LAV NRW R, Gerichte Rep 139. Nr. 14 Bl. 013-027); and from known birth locations of Thalidomide Trust beneficiaries. It is the case that thalidomide children were born in countries such as France (1 report), East Germany (possibly 80+) and the USA where the drug was never licensed. This is because of people (including doctors) bringing the drug in from countries where it was available, samples distributed for marketing purposes, and even mothers giving birth in a different country from the one where they were provided with the drug (2 of these known in USA).

[32] Stephens, T., Brynner, R, *Dark Remedy; the impact of Thalidomide and its revival as a vital medicine* (New York: Perseus, 2001) p. 37.

number of adults affected could well have been in the order of half a million, possibly more.[33]

The toll on parents and families

In the UK and Germany, many of the couples who had thalidomide children ended up divorcing. This is a sad but common consequence of attempting to bring up children with chronic illnesses or disabilities. Even more seriously, a number of parents committed suicide. One UK thalidomider spoke of this experience and its consequences:

> *I grew up in a home for deaf children. When I was 18 months old my mother killed herself because of my disabilities, and my father could not cope with bringing up both my older brother and me.*[34]

Other parents went 'off the rails' in different ways, with alcohol or gambling, or by embarking on business activities that were clearly ill-conceived and therefore doomed from the start. Many siblings of survivors never came to terms with the extra attention given to their thalidomide brothers or sisters, or with the money that ultimately became available to them. It is clear, too, that many families were deeply ashamed of their affected children: some thalidomiders, both in UK and elsewhere, were kept hidden by their families. One Scottish survivor said her father built an eight-foot wall around their back garden, so the neighbours could not see her when she went out to play.[35] From Germany, Claudia Schmidt-Herterich recalls:

> *When I was a member of the 'youth board' of the Thalidomide Society of North-Rhine Westphalia 1980/1981 we got a phone call from inhabitants of a village in the area. Those people told us that in their neighbourhood lived a thalidomider. Nobody has ever seen him on the street, in a school or anywhere, but they have observed a boy sometimes in the dark in the garden or at a window. He limped, had short arms and looked very deformed. They asked us to visit the neighbours to check on it. You can*

[33] Daemmrich, A., 'A Tale of Two Experts: Thalidomide and Political Engagement in the United States and Germany', *Social History of Medicine* 15, No. 1 (2002), pp. 137-158; Eriksson, T, Bjorkman, S. and Hoglund, P., 'Clinical pharmacology of Thalidomide', *European Journal of Clinical Pharmacology* 27 (2001): 365-376.

[34] Female, during visit by Martin Johnson, 29 January 2001.

[35] Female thalidomider (now deceased), ref. 146, in conversations with Martin Johnson concluding with visit on 1 September 2008.

imagine that this was not very easy for us. How should we go there and ring the bell? What reason should we come up with?...

In the end, as I knew that village very well from my childhood, I went there and decided in advance to be honest and straight. I met a man about 20 years old and told him that we think that somebody lives here who looks like me and we would like to visit him as volunteers. He was alone (without the parents) at home and let me in. What I saw there, I will never forget.

We went into a room with a bed by the wall, dark windows and there in the bed lay a young man. He was not able to communicate with me and was of course full of fear as he saw me, a stranger looking like him. The brother felt very ashamed but on the other hand very, very relieved, at least this was my impression. The man in the bed was totally neglected, was very weak, because – so I was told – he rarely stands up, because one leg is much shorter than the other. The brother said that the parents feel very ashamed and did not want the others to know and see that they have such a deformed child.

You can imagine how horrified I was. I left the household after 30 minutes, phoned the department of social help and they – I heard later – went into the household with the police, got the man out and after getting medical help moved him to a home for disabled people. Until now, I still have contact with the brother of the thalidomider. The thalidomider lives in a home still, is mentally and psychologically quite affected, though he seems to feel well in his surroundings, but he still avoids going out when it is bright and sunny outside...[36]

More seriously still, though, a significant number of thalidomide children were subjected to sexual, physical or financial abuse – sometimes all three. Here is a selection of reports from the records of the UK Thalidomide Trust:

When I was eight, one of the helpers in the [church-run] children's home sexually abused me. I told the person in charge, but she did not believe me, and I was punished for being a

[36] Email from Claudia Schmidt-Herterich to Martin Johnson, 17 December 2011, 18:15.

naughty girl, making up a story like that. I think I became more upset about being disbelieved than I was about the abuse.[37]

Another reported:

My father started abusing me. One night, I saw my sister watching through the bedroom door. I have never been able to forgive her for not telling anyone what she saw.[38]

He was not the only one. A female thalidomider told the Thalidomide Trust:

My father started having sex with me when I was 10. I tried telling my mother, but she refused to believe me, so it kept on happening until I was 15, when I ran away from home.[39]

These stories are representative of many similar incidents. Despite several reports of sexual abuse of thalidomide children, there have never been any cases of perpetrators brought to trial. This could be because of the particular difficulty these children had of getting anyone to believe that there were paedophile adults who preyed upon children with such severe disabilities. One case illustrates this well: 13-year old Louise Mason was raped in the care home she lived in by a much older boy. Her cries of protest during the rape were ignored by a nearby staff member, and when she reported the attack, she was seen by the doctor, who went on to tell her father that she was confused and possibly having her first period. He did not bother to look for the obvious evidence that would show what had taken place.[40]

These stories, coupled with the far more widespread problems of financial exploitation once the children received their first settlement funds, together with other physical and mental abuses, illustrate some of the appalling secondary consequences of this disaster. But it is important to underscore that thalidomide injuries had effects that went not only into childhood, but also into adolescence, young adulthood and beyond. At the age of fifty, for example, around half of all survivors were coping with chronic pain, largely as a result of the

[37] Female thalidomider, four-limb deficient (now deceased), ref. 136, September 2000.

[38] Male thalidomider, severe lower-limb damage (now deceased), ref. 62, in conversation with Martin Johnson during visit, 18 December 2003.

[39] Female thalidomider, severe upper-limb damage, in conversation with Martin Johnson during visit 1 September 2005.

[40] Louise Medus-Mansell, *No Hands to Hold and No Legs to Dance On; a Thalidomide Survivors Tale* (Accent Press, 2009) pp. 78-79. This account has been verified by the author(s) with other thalidomide survivors who were resident in the same establishment at the time.

challenges of living with missing or damaged limbs.[41] For many, their bodies are deteriorating far faster than other people of their age. At least a quarter are coping with emergent neurological problems, tingling, numbness, and pain in their affected limbs. Such a person may be holding a cup, for instance, and the next thing they know is it has fallen to the floor and broken, because of the numbness in their hand. For these survivors, the thalidomide catastrophe is still slowly unfolding in their day-to-day lives. The damage to their bodies is not yet finished.

Could the catastrophe have been avoided or averted?

Figure 3: UK Thalidomide Births, January 1958 - May 1965.

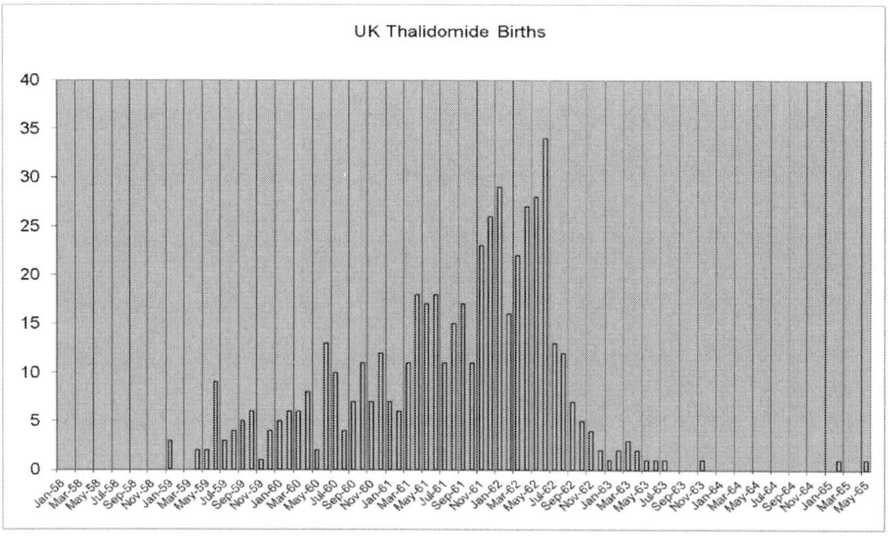

Source: Thalidomide Trust records of birthdates.

Figure 3 illustrates the effects of the rapid increase in sales of thalidomide in the UK in the late 1950s and early 1960s on births of affected children. Two trends are particularly significant. First, the number of recorded thalidomide births reached its peak in June 1962, twice as many as a year earlier, and about four times as many as two years earlier. The second trend has to do with the rapid fall in the number of thalidomide births during the summer of 1962. By August,

41 Martin Johnson (2007) 'Integrating health information: A case study of a health information service for Thalidomide Survivors', *Medical Informatics and the Internet in Medicine* March 2007; 32(1): 27-33.

about nine months after the news of the birth defect risks went public leading to the withdrawal of the drug from sales in November 1961, the number of births recorded decreased dramatically. Taken together, these two trends suggest strongly that earlier withdrawal of the drug would have avoided a large amount of damage to babies through thalidomide, whether through causing miscarriage or stillbirth or through causing birth defects. Each delay in withdrawal of the drug from sale, then, had major and severe consequences.

Two dates in particular are worth highlighting in this regard. First, all of this could have been avoided in the first place, at least in some countries: for instance, the drug was released in the UK in April 1958 despite a public report three months earlier advising that it affected the thyroid gland – a very strong contraindication for use during pregnancy. Had that warning been heeded, the thalidomide catastrophe in Britain could have been averted. But thalidomide should surely have been withdrawn from sale at the latest by the second key date, 14 July 1961, when, in response to the vast number of serious complaints about the drug, Heinrich Mückter told his staff that '...if I were a doctor, I would not prescribe Contergan any more. Gentlemen, I warn you, I will not repeat what has already been said before. I see great dangers.'[42] Yet, he allowed the sales to continue unchecked. This was catastrophic: indeed, if the drug had been withdrawn then rather than four months later (after Professor Widukind Lenz told managers at Chemie Grünenthal on 16 November 1961 that he had strong evidence to suggest that the company's thalidomide-based drugs were causing the epidemic of birth defects then happening throughout Germany), more than 25% of the babies who were in fact ultimately affected would have been saved. What is more, in between these two dates, Chemie Grünenthal received approximately 2,500 warnings of adverse side effects, mainly from doctors who had prescribed the drug – or even used it to treat their own wives – all of which were effectively ignored.

But there were indications even earlier that thalidomide was dangerous, and which should have sent alarm bells ringing. The Distillers Company, which eventually obtained a licence for manufacture and sale of the drug in the UK, had thalidomide tested by two expert pharmacologists, who published their findings in the *British Medical Journal* on 11 January 1958. They reported that it suppressed

[42] Quoted in Henning Sjöström, Robert Nilsson, *Thalidomide and the power of the drug companies* (Harmondsworth: Penguin, 1972) p. 88.

the thyroid gland. Their key conclusion was: 'In the meantime, therefore, it would seem unjustifiable to use the drug for long-term sedative or hypnotic therapy...' (which, of course, was the precise target market for the drug). In any event, the anti-thyroid effects should have meant it would be kept away from pregnant women.[43] Seven months later, in August 1958, trials of the drug undertaken by prospective American licensee Smith Kline & French resulted in the birth of a clearly damaged child. There is no direct evidence that the American firm reported this to Chemie Grünenthal, although there must have been a contractual obligation to do so. Whether that happened or not, though, this was clearly one of the reasons that the American company, which had initially been quite enthusiastic about taking up Grünenthal's offer of a licence to distribute it in the USA, decided instead to turn it down.[44]

The significance of all of this cannot be exaggerated: acting on either of these reports would have saved nearly all the children eventually affected by thalidomide. What is more, acting on two reports of birth defect risks nearly a year later from a Dr. Kreideweiß in April 1959 (three thalidomide birth defect cases reported), or Professor Riemschneider in June 1959 (who had induced birth defects in amphibians while testing thalidomide) would have saved around 90% of the victims.[45]

But, in the meantime, sales of the drug had taken off, and Grünenthal (along with its licensees) began to enjoy large and growing profits, so much so that the company ignored any evidence of thalidomide's devastating effects, even if that evidence came from within. For instance, in November 1959, an internal report prepared for the German company's directors informed them of research showing that drug 'K17' (their designation for thalidomide in trials) was likely to have a mechanism of action of a type that was well-known to cause

43 J. McC. Murdoch, G.D. Campbell (1958) 'Antithyroid activity of N-Phthalyl Glutamic Acid Imide (K 17)', *BMJ* (11 January 1958), p. 84. This is dealt with more fully in Chapter 5.

44 See claim filed 9 August 2012 in Philadelphia County Court of Common pleas, which indicates documentary evidence of testing by Smith, Kline and French in 1956 showed thalidomide useless as a sedative, and one, possibly two babies with birth defects born to women in August 1958 among a group of 875 people who took the drug during testing: *http://www.hbsslaw.com/resources/newsroom/hagens-berman-files-new-lawsuit-on-behalf-of-11-alleged-us-thalidomide-victims* <viewed 13 March 2013>. See also Gemballa, *Der dreifache Skandal; 30 Jahre nach Contergan Eine Dokumentation,* Luchterhand Literaturverlag GmbH, Hamburg (1993), pp. 46-47.

45 Prof. Dr. Ralph Riemschneider (2004) 'Thalidomide A remedy with two faces', *The BWW Society, the Institute for the Advancement of Positive Global Solutions* (Nov/Dec Issue 2004).

severe birth defects.[46] Reports from outside the firm were similarly ignored. In April 1961, in one of a series of monthly meetings to consider what should be done about the flood of warnings coming in about the drug, Grünenthal staff specifically discussed the possible relationship between the action of K17 and Aminopterin, as published by Thiersch in 1952 ('Therapeutic Abortions with a Folic Acid Antagonist'). They decided to do nothing, however.[47]

Even at that late stage in spring 1961, half the children eventually affected by the drug would have been saved had it been withdrawn then. What is more, a month after the Grünenthal staff meeting just mentioned, in May 1961, Distillers were warned by Dr. William McBride, a gynaecologist and obstetrician in Sydney, of his suspicions that the drug had been causing birth defects in his patients. Even then, just six months before withdrawal, 46% of the victims could have been saved. The final four-month delay, following Heinrich Mückter's warning to the Grünenthal staff, led to at least 460 UK thalidomide survivors and 4,600 survivors worldwide being affected. And of course, the number of survivors can be multiplied by as much as 10 to arrive at an estimate of the numbers destroyed in the womb or stillborn.

In other words, there were early, repeated and credible warnings that thalidomide could have been reasonably expected to pose the dangers it in fact exhibited. Yet Chemie Grünenthal refused to withdraw it until November 1961. The reluctance shown by the company probably involved a few factors, most notably that by the time thalidomide was introduced, the company's profits from its other products had declined sharply as a result of competition. Thalidomide offered an ever more lucrative route out of this profit squeeze. What is more, company managers had also managed to escape censure or litigation over at least two earlier products which had proved very risky, possibly causing a number of deaths, so they may have felt able to overcome the thalidomide problem in a similar way. And it is especially striking that the drug did not simply go away after November 1961. For one thing, as indicated in Figure 3, the withdrawal of thalidomide

46 Monthly report by Dr. Michael November 1959 (Gerichte Rep 139 No 21 157) LA NRW Duisburg: Dr. Michaels wrote that a Dr. Wowalka had been studying the mechanism of action of K17, and considered it to be an anti-glutamic acid action which was potentially teratogenic.

47 Extract from a travel report of Dr. Michael of Chemie Grünenthal from 5 April 1961 that he presented and put up for discussion in Stolberg – the discussion included reference to possible antivitamin action of K17, with explicit reference to the 1952 work by Thiersch. Leitende Oberstaatsanwalt be idem Landgericht Aachen, 'Anklage gegen Wirtz u.a. Contergan-Verfahren', 10 March 1967, vol. I, p. 463.

from sale slowed, but did not entirely stop, the incidence of births of survivors: in the UK, there are registered thalidomiders born as late as 1965, an indication of just how difficult it is to withdraw a drug from the public entirely. And this pattern would have occurred in other markets as well. What is more, Grünenthal staff played a leading role in attempting to find new uses for thalidomide after November 1961 – leprosy and cancer treatments were their early objectives. This in turn triggered the proliferation of the drug in Latin America, leading to a second wave of the thalidomide catastrophe that began in Brazil in the early 1970s. And it has yet to end.

The right to life

Countless tens of thousands of babies were denied their right to life while still inside their mother's wombs because of the Grünenthal lie that thalidomide was 'safe for pregnant women' rather than the dangerous neurotoxin the company's managers really knew it to be. Moreover, unknown numbers, certainly hundreds if not thousands, were put to death by the midwives and doctors attending their births, arbitrarily denying them what could have been a full life. The massive public support for Suzanne van der Put's acquittal of murder in Belgium demonstrates that denying disabled babies their right to life was widely approved of in society, and surely this was not a belief held just by Belgians alone.

Then there is the fact that compensation in all the countries where it was paid was limited to only those children who survived long enough – a mere 25% or so of those who survived birth and into their teenage years. For thousands and thousands of children maimed and eventually killed by the effects of this drug, all of whom had names and families, there has never been any compensation; never anyone convicted in respect of their deaths; never any public enquiry to ascertain who they were, what happened to them or how the catastrophe was caused. The guilt of the manufacturers and distributors is plain to see, as is also the guilt of those governments which failed to ensure the safety of their own people with proper drug controls. And before we accept the usual excuse here that such controls would have required an awareness of the risks and the science involved that went beyond the standards of the time, it must be remembered that countries which did deny or significantly restrict the introduction of thalidomide included not only the USA, but also Turkey, East Germany and France. Moreover, in Portugal and Austria, regulators raised serious questions about the drug, which in Austria led to a ban on over-the-counter sales.

From Christmas Day 1956 in the town of Stolberg, Germany, where Chemie Grünenthal was located, through to 9 December 2010 in Maranhäo, Brazil, children have been born damaged by thalidomide. It is likely that for each thalidomide child who has survived to adulthood, probably three more will have died on the way, not living long enough to be registered in national compensation schemes. And for those four, up to another ten babies will have been destroyed in the womb. The selling ground for these tablets seems to have shifted away from Europe, North America, Australia and Japan to the developing world, impelled by an unending drive by medical researchers to find positive applications for it, despite the lack of unequivocal evidence that thalidomide has ever cured any cancer or any other serious disease after more than 50 years of human experiments.

The toll of the catastrophe has clearly been enormous, and is ongoing. And there is a very real question about when it will stop, which we will take up again later in the book. But what we want to do before that is to explore another set of questions:

- How did it start?
- Why and how did it continue even in spite of mounting evidence of the destruction inflicted by the drug?
- Why and how has no one been held to account for the disaster?
- And, significantly, what has been – and still needs to be – done to compensate the victims?

Figure 4: Countries of known thalidomide births.

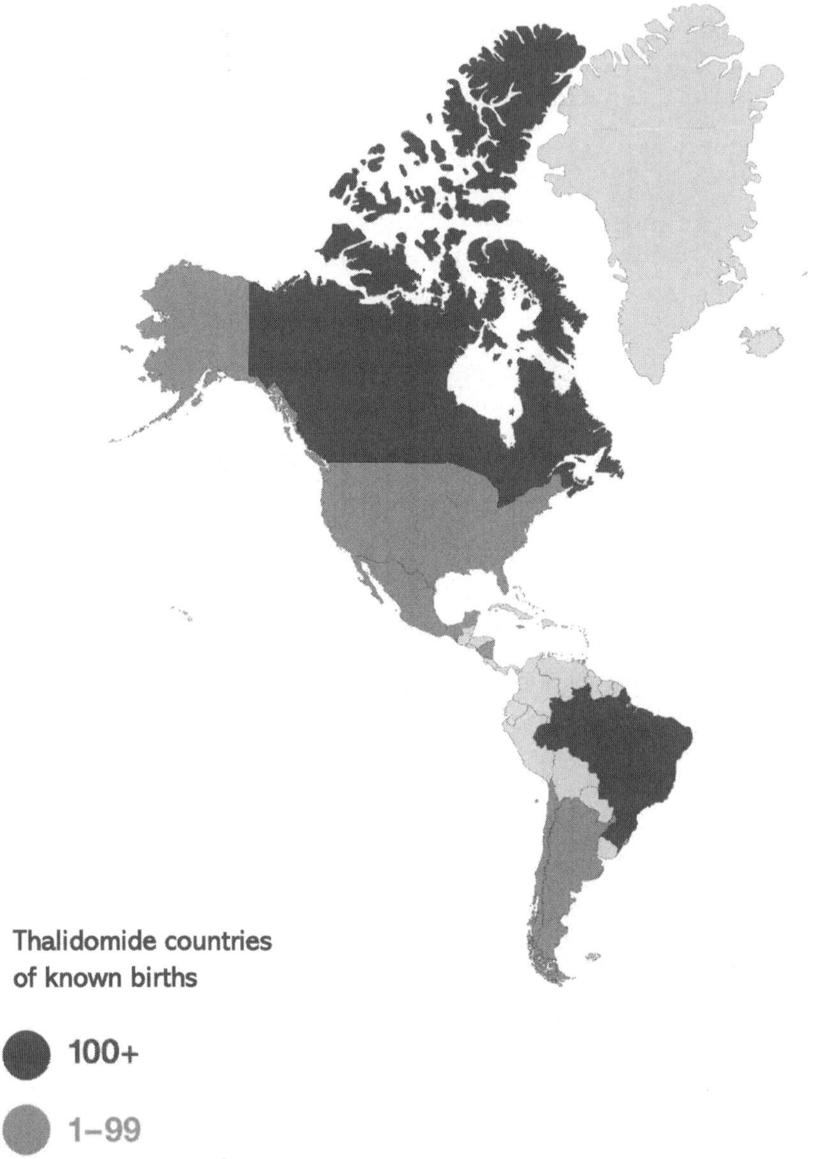

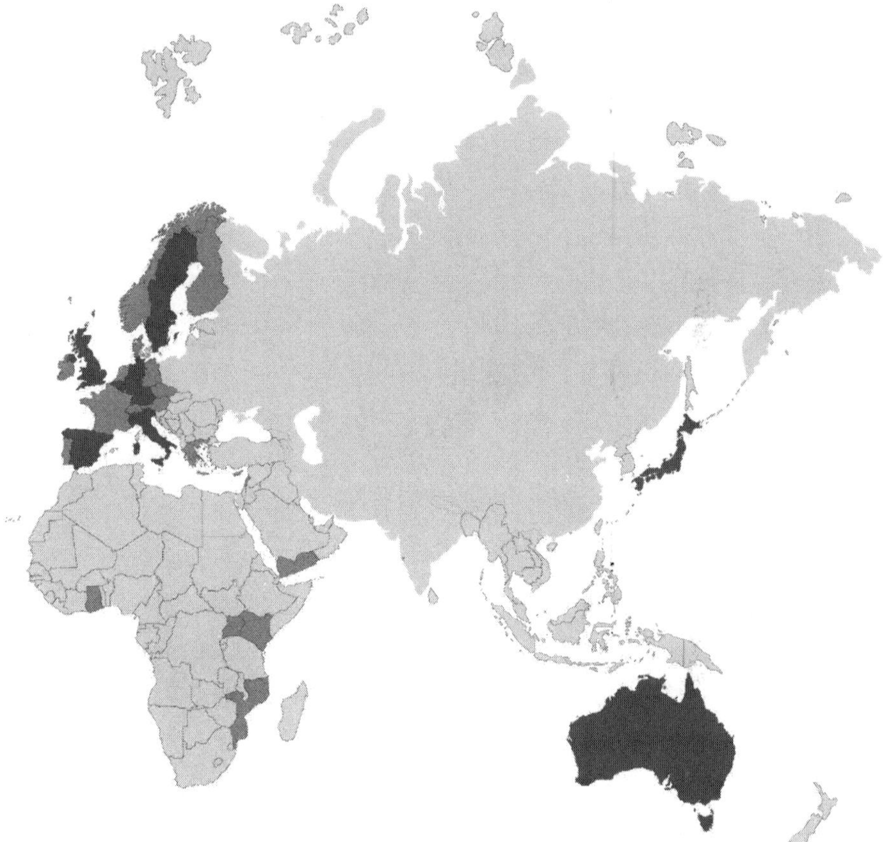

Figure 5: Frederic Sanders b. April 1962 d. February 1963
with mother, Gertrud, and sister, Christine.
Nobody in Fredric's family ever met anyone in the same situation, and, after Frederic's death, stopped fighting for compensation or relief. Frederic's mother suffered from poor mental health for the rest of her life after Frederic's death.

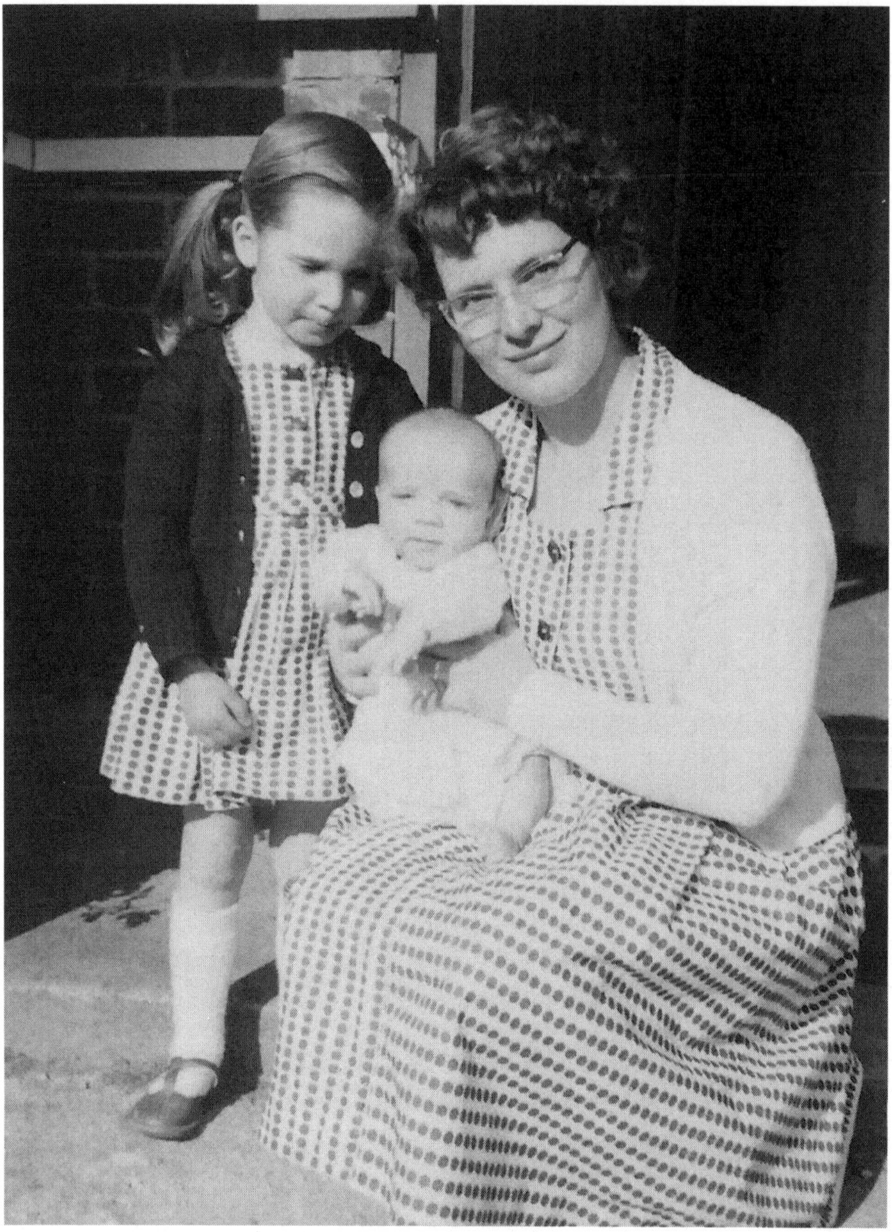

© Thalidomide Society on behalf of the copyright holder

Chapter Two

Setting the Scene

Establishing networks and routines in National Socialist Germany.

WHERE CAN WE FIND THE ORIGINS of thalidomide and the disaster it unleashed? Some would situate the beginnings in the Third Reich, which is not as far-fetched as it perhaps sounds. After all, there have been suggestions from time to time that thalidomide may have been synthesised for the first time in Nazi-dominated Europe, perhaps, as has been surmised by one of the co-authors of this book, in connection with the development and testing of nerve gases (Tabun and Sarin) and of nerve gas antidotes to counteract their effects.[48] Yet, although there are plausible grounds for the speculation about the drug's connection to chemical warfare (which we consider later in this chapter), there is no smoking gun in the documentary evidence that would establish conclusively that thalidomide originated during the National Socialist period. In fact, although one journalist has claimed to have found a document from 1944 allegedly proving the drug's Nazi origins,[49] no one has been able to verify the reliability or even the existence of that document or any other dating from the Nazi period on thalidomide. The plain truth therefore is this: we just do not know.

Still, regardless of this lack of firm evidence that thalidomide was first made in the Nazi period, it is also a fact that the origins and unfolding of the thalidomide disaster cannot be understood without

[48] Daniel Foggo, 'Thalidomide "was created by the Nazis"', *The Sunday Times* (8 February 2009), available at: *http://www.thesundaytimes.co.uk/sto/style/living/Health/article148972.ece* <viewed 8 June 2015>.

[49] *Ibid.*

consideration of aspects of the history of the German pharmaceuticals industry, in particular as it developed in the National Socialist period. It was then that the networks of people and organisations were formed that had direct bearing on the drug's destructive impact from the 1950s onwards. And it was then that patterns of behaviour emerged within these networks that would shape the widespread deployment of thalidomide, its continued sale in the face of mounting evidence of its toxicity and effects on pregnant women, and the extraordinary efforts devoted to evading responsibility for the human costs of the drug.

The many faces of the German pharmaceuticals industry

The first artificial dyestuffs were synthesised in England in 1856, and the origins of the modern chemicals industry are therefore in Britain and France, not in one of what were then the still disunited states of the German area. Still, by the time the German Empire was proclaimed in the Hall of Mirrors at Versailles in 1871, the new country's firms, many of them founded in the 1860s, were well on the way to making Germany the undisputed world leader in the organic chemicals industry. In fact, by 1913, led by companies like BASF, Bayer, Agfa and Meister Lucius and Brüning (with its primary factory at Hoechst, which will be the designation used for the company from now on), Germany controlled nearly 90% of world trade in synthetic dyestuffs and other organic chemicals. The absolutely dominant international position was in part the result of product, process and organisational innovation in key firms: for instance, BASF created the world's first dedicated modern industrial laboratory, facilitating an ever-growing outpouring of inventions, and the other major German firms soon followed suit. But an important underpinning enabling the firms' dominance came from the support structure put in place by the new German national government, and even more importantly by the federal states that made up the new country. The federal government enacted an innovative patent law in 1877 that enabled protection of processes rather than products, thus spurring chemical innovation. The federal states in turn provided excellent universities where the professoriate carried out important research that often complemented that done in the industrial laboratories; but, even more importantly, the universities trained the chemists needed by industry.[50]

Even as the major chemical firms grew into international forces to be reckoned with by the late 19th century, many of them began seeking to deploy the skills they had developed in dealing with components of coal tar to branch out into synthesis and production of pharmaceuticals, although BASF shied away from the area as too risky. As was the case with coal-tar dyes, new synthetic pharmaceuticals not only replaced natural materials such as plant extracts that were often difficult to obtain, certainly in any standard form; they also allowed for the creation of entirely new products for which there were no natural analogues. And for some companies such as Bayer and Hoechst, the foray into the new field was a particularly lucrative business. A chemist at Bayer, for instance, synthesised pure acetylsalicylic acid for the first time in 1897, which under its trade name 'Aspirin' proved to be one of the most successful medicines of all time.[51]

Again, connections with German universities were important in this development, especially because many of them were extremely strong not just in chemistry, but also in biology and medicine. Here, the pioneering work in bacteriology done by Robert Koch and scientists such as Paul Ehrlich in Koch's Institute for Infectious Diseases led not only to the isolation of the bacteria that cause diseases such as tuberculosis, but also to the development of key pharmaceutical products, including vaccines and specialist medicines. Ehrlich, for instance, was responsible for the synthesis of the drug Salvarsan, introduced into the market in 1910 as the first 'magic bullet' that could cure syphilis without harming the patient, a product and event which also 'marked the beginning of targeted chemotherapy'.[52]

50 A brief overview of the early history of the German chemical industry is in Raymond G. Stokes, *Divide and Prosper: The Heirs to IG Farben under Allied Authority, 1945-1951* (Berkeley: University of California Press, 1988); paperback edition with new forward (Udderfield: Hexagon Press, 2009), pp. 4-11. On BASF as the first dedicated industrial laboratory, see Ernst Homburg, 'The Emergence of research laboratories in the dyestuffs industry, 1870-1900', *British Journal for the History of Science* 25 (1992): 91-111.

51 'Aspirin', Royal Society for Chemistry, 2003, at: *www.rsc.org/learn-chemistry/content/filerepository/CMP/.../Aspirin.pdf* <viewed 15 June 2015>; also, 'A History of Aspirin', *Clinical Pharmacist* (September 2014), Vol 6, No 7 *http://www.pharmaceutical-journal.com/publications/previous-issues/cp-september-2014/a-history-of-aspirin/20066661.article* <viewed 15 June 2015>.

52 On Koch's life and work, see Thomas D. Brock, *Robert Koch: A life in medicine and bacteriology* (Berlin: Springer, 1988); quotation from: 'Salvarsan', *Chemical and Engineering News* 83 (20 June 2005), available at: *http://pubs.acs.org/cen/coverstory/83/8325/8325salvarsan.html* <viewed 9 June 2015>.

Such work at German universities and university-level institutes complemented that done by firms in the country's chemical industry, but it also formed the basis of close cooperation in the development, and in particular the commercialisation, of new drugs and therapies. One particularly striking example of this interpenetration of science, medicine and industry – and of the pitfalls and problems that it could lead to – was the Behring-Werke, which was founded in Marburg in 1904. This laboratory and manufacturing facility, which combined scientific research with extensive commercial operations, was the brainchild of Emil von Behring, a Marburg University professor who established it using the prize money from his 1901 Nobel Prize in Medicine (which he won for his development of serum therapy for diphtheria, much of the research for which was done in Koch's Institute in the 1890s). Von Behring also used funding from Hoechst to finance some of his ongoing research, with the chemical firm commercialising key aspects of it. The Behring-Werke moved to much larger premises in nearby Marbach in 1913 and flourished even after relations with Hoechst became strained in the years that followed and especially in the aftermath of von Behring's death as a result of a lung infection in 1917.[53]

But the company did not stay independent for very long after von Behring died, in part because it was so successful. Not long after IG Farbenindustrie AG was formed in 1925 as a conglomerate that included the largest German chemical firms (including BASF, Hoechst and Bayer), the Behring-Werke became a wholly owned subsidiary of the new chemical giant and was eventually assigned, along with Hoechst and a few others in the middle Rhine region, to the IG Farben Maingau Works Group, although relations with the main Hoechst factory continued to be strained because a large proportion of the Group's pharmaceutical production was assigned to the Behring-Werke.[54] During the Third Reich, the Behring-Werke's activities were as crucial to the Wehrmacht as they were morally problematic. The utter

[53] On von Behring's research and work at the Koch Institute: *http://www.nobelprize.org/nobel_prizes/medicine/laureates/1901/behring-article.html* <viewed 9 June 2015>; on von Behring and the Behring-Werke through 1917: *https://www.uni-marburg.de/fb20/evbb/behring-digital/leben-werk/behringwerke* <viewed 9 June 2015>; on relations between von Behring and the Behring-Werke and Hoechst, Derek S. Linton, *Emil von Behring: Infectious disease, immunology, serum therapy* (Philadelphia: American Philosophical Society, 2005) p. 101.

[54] Stephan Lindner, *Inside IG Farben: Hoechst during the Third Reich* (Cambridge/NY: Cambridge University Press, 2008) passim, esp. pp. 55, 57, 117.

reliance of the armed forces on the Behring-Werke is evident from just a few statistics: the works and its related factories supplied 100% of the army's demand for sera for treatment of a number of different diseases, and in addition, it and the rest of IG Farben supplied some 55% of the army's pharmaceutical needs.[55] The IG subsidiary's moral bankruptcy, however, is just as obvious. Managing Director Albert Demnitz demonstrated this in a particularly appalling way in January 1940 at a meeting at the Behring-Werke, insisting to fellow scientists that 'experiments on humans are to be strived for' so as to enable the further development of medicines in service of the war effort. Actions were as good as Demnitz's word: the Behring-Werke, other parts of IG Farben, and other pharmaceutical firms and research institutes participated actively, for instance, in human experiments to develop medical preparations to combat typhus at the Buchenwald concentration camp,[56] a crime we will revisit later in the chapter.

At this point, though, it is important to stress that the history of the Behring-Werke illustrates graphically three key tensions and relationships that have shaped the development of the German chemical and pharmaceuticals industries. The first was that between academia and private-sector firms (often mediated, informed or guided by the state and its ideology and policies, in particular in times of war). The second key tension was between, on the one hand, excellence in the service of good and, on the other hand, scientific excellence deployed in callous and inhumane ways, in particular – but not exclusively – in the Nazi era. These first two relationships were especially prominent in regard to the large-scale firms that are well known, companies such as BASF, Bayer and Hoechst. But there is a third set of tensions/relationships that have shaped the history of the chemical and pharmaceutical industries in Germany, particularly the pharmaceuticals: the interconnections between the small number of prominent large-scale firms and the raft of much smaller ones. It is a relationship we know much less about than the other two, despite the fact that firms outside of IG Farben supplied fully 45% of the Wehrmacht's pharmaceutical requirements during the war. In any case, though, it is a relationship that appears to have been

55 See graph reproduced from an investigation of IG Farben conducted in autumn 1945 by the Office of US Military Government in Germany (OMGUS) in OMGUS, *Die Ermittlung gegen die IG Farbenindustrie AG September 1945* (Nördlingen: Franz Greno, 1986) p. 348.

56 Thomas Werther, '"Anzustreben sind Versuche am Menschen…": Ein kurzer Beitrag zur Geschichte der Marburger Behringwerke', Geschichtswerkstatt Marburg e.V., available at: *http://www.geschichtswerkstatt-marburg.de/projekte/behrng.php* <viewed 12 June 2015>.

mediated, at least in part, by university professors and scientists, and also by key figures with contacts in both camps, as we shall see in our exploration of the networks and patterns of behaviour constructed during the Third Reich, all of which set the stage for the founding of Chemie Grünenthal in 1946.

Networks and nodes: pharmaceuticals in the Nazi era

The network has become a common metaphor in scholarly and popular discourse about dynamic interactions among humans, organisations and technological systems over time, in particular in the history of science, technology and medicine, and in business history. This is no doubt in part because of the early and effective use of the metaphor in Thomas Parke Hughes's comparative study from 1983 of the development of the electrical power industry in the United States, the United Kingdom and Germany from 1880-1930, *Networks of Power*.[57] More recently, scholarly and popular literature, again in particular in history of science, technology and medicine, but also in business history, has focused not just on networks, but even more keenly on the nodes within them, i.e. the key points in a network where a number of pathways intersect. A node can of course be a person, an organisation or a thing, or some combination of all three, but in socio-technical networks, people are often key. Some historians, for instance, use the notion of a 'Big Linker' in this context.[58] A good example is Fritz Haber, the academic physical chemist with tight links to industry and government that resulted in enormous influence and impact, not least through his work on synthetic nitrates (produced via the Haber-Bosch process, which enabled large-scale production of artificial fertilisers and also ammunition for the German war effort between 1914 and 1918) and on the development of poison gases, also during the First World War.[59] For the prehistory of thalidomide in the Nazi era there were three Big Linkers, Werner Schulemann, Heinrich Mückter and Otto Ambros, all

[57] Thomas Parke Hughes, *Networks of Power: Electrification in Western Society, 1880-1930* (Baltimore: Johns Hopkins University Press, 1983).

[58] See, for instance, the use of the term in Gerhard Schnyder and John F. Wilson, 'The structure of networks: The transformation of UK business, 1904-2010)', p. 55, in Thomas David and Gerarda Westerhuis, eds., *The Power of Corporate Networks: A Comparative and Historical Perspective* (New York/Abingdon: Routledge, 2014).

[59] For the definitive biography of Haber, see Margit Szöllösi-Janze, *Fritz Haber 1868-1934. Eine Biographie* (Munich: CH Beck, 1998).

of whom eventually converged on the critical artefactual node which connected all of these networks: thalidomide.

WERNER SCHULEMANN (1888-1975)[60]

Werner Schulemann was a highly qualified chemist and medical doctor who excelled at pharmaceutical invention, and his career involved a classic trajectory featuring intensive academic-industry interaction, political involvement and commercialisation of new drugs that led to substantial personal wealth. He earned a doctorate in chemistry in 1913 and then completed his degree as a medical doctor the following year, before working during the 1914-1918 war as a surgeon. His move from academic research to medical practice led eventually to undertaking commercially relevant pharmaceutical development at the end of the war, when he took a position in the research department of Bayer AG in Wuppertal-Elberfeld. There his career flourished, especially after Bayer, along with BASF, Hoechst and a number of other chemical firms in Germany (including the Behring-Werke) became a part of the IG Farben chemical conglomerate. By 1931, he was the director of the department of pharmaceutical synthesis. His research there on chemotherapeutic treatments for malaria resulted in medicines that 'count among the most important results of pharmaceutical research in the 20th century', and his work was duly recognised nationally and internationally. In 1928, he and his two co-inventors were awarded the prestigious Emil-Fischer Memorial Medal of the German Chemical Society. Schulemann was also awarded the Mary Kingsley medal (of the Liverpool School of Tropical Medicine) in 1938 for his achievements in developing synthetic antimalarials.[61] In recognition of this same work on antimalarials, he was nominated in 1934 and 1935 for a Nobel Prize in physiology or medicine.[62] And his scientific achievements were not restricted to this field: he also worked fruitfully during his career as a Bayer researcher

60 For more on Schulemann's career, see Marion A. Hulverscheidt, 'The scientist-entrepreneur, or financing in pharmaceutical researcg: A portrait of the malariologist Werner Schulemann, 1888-1975', pp. 121-148 in Viviane Quirke and Judy Slinn, eds, *Perspectives on twentieth-century pharmaceuticals* (Oxford: Peter Lang, 2010).

61 'Local News', *BMJ* (31 December 1938) pp. 1386-1387.

62 See *http://www.nobelprize.org/nomination/archive/show_people.php?id=8247* <viewed 7 February 2016>.

on successful development of sleeping pills, disinfectants and local anaesthetics.[63]

But he was also developing other, less savoury, interests and connections while at Bayer. In 1933, after the National Socialist seizure of power, he became a member of the SA, the party's storm trooper regiment, although he was prevented from joining the party itself until 1937, when a 1933 Nazi policy preventing new members from joining the party was lifted. Shortly before Schulemann joined the Nazi party, he fell out with his line manager at IG Farben and was dismissed, although retained on full pay. Still only in his late forties, Schulemann understandably cast about for a new job, this time deciding to make the move back to academe from business, and he applied for a professorship at the University of Bonn. The appointment process was byzantine, and Schulemann's political connections had some impact here, although apparently not always in his favour. It all ended in 1938 with his appointment to the Chair of Pharmacology and Toxicology in the medical faculty at the University of Bonn. Regardless of the role of his connections and convictions in the appointment, Schulemann was unabashed in his public display of them: he upset a number of other members of the medical faculty by delivering his inaugural lecture not in academic dress, but instead in his SA uniform.[64]

Schulemann continued his research work on antimalarials at the University of Bonn during the Second World War, but he also worked in chemical warfare research, both with phosgene and with 'new chemical weapons' (i.e. nerve agents), focusing in particular on development of antidotes to minimise damage from them, and he was implicated in experiments on prisoners. Funded by the German Research Foundation, Schulemann also did research on typhus and other infectious diseases.[65] From at least 1937 onwards, he is known to have directed human tests for malaria research using paralysed people and soldiers in field hospitals.[66] As a result of this research activity and his membership in the Nazi party and the SA, Schulemann was suspended from his post at the university by Allied authorities after the

63 Holldorf, August W., 'Schulemann, Werner', *Neue Deutsche Biographie* 23 (2007), S. 675-676 [Onlinefassung]; at: *http://www.deutsche-biographie.de/ppn117160164.html* <viewed 9 June 2015>.

64 Eckart W.U. (Ed.), *Man, medicine, and the state* (Stuttgart: Steiner, 2006) pp. 232-235. Ralf Forsbach, *Die medizinische Fakultät der Universität Bonn im 'Dritten Reich'* (Munich: Oldenbourg, 2006) pp. 100-103.

65 Ralf Forsbach, *Die medizinische Fakultät der Universität Bonn im 'Dritten Reich'*, pp. 471-474.

66 Eckart W.U. (Ed.), *Man, medicine, and the state*, p. 233.

war as part of the denazification process, although he was quietly reinstated in 1949/50. Thereafter, his period of disgrace was discreetly expunged from the record, and he then continued working at the University of Bonn until his retirement in 1958 at the age of 70.[67]

Schulemann's career, at times brilliant and at times – especially during the Nazi period, but also at other times – highly problematic, was connected, directly and indirectly, in a number of ways with the origins and unfolding of the thalidomide disaster. First of all, as will become increasingly evident later in this and subsequent chapters, Schulemann's close and longstanding working relationships with a number of key firms in the pharmaceuticals industry, in particular Bayer/IG Farben and Schering, were important, and he served as a personal and professional link between these firms and smaller ones, including eventually Chemie Grünenthal. Second, it is highly significant that thalidomide is closely related chemically to the classes of compounds on which much of Schulemann's research and patent activity focused, i.e. quinine, synthetic antimalarials and glutamic acid derivatives.[68] This experience is highly relevant because of a third, even more important, connection to thalidomide: as a recently appointed professor, Schulemann helped train Dr. Heinrich Mückter, the later chief scientist at Chemie Grünenthal, as a medical doctor at the University of Bonn between 1938 and 1940, and taught him again immediately after the war in the degree programme in pharmacology that Mückter completed even as he took up Grünenthal's chief scientist position in 1946.[69] Mückter regarded Schulemann as a most supportive and highly respected friend in later years. He kept a photograph on the wall of his study at home, which showed him with Schulemann and two other prominent professors he had studied with. Among those three teachers, Mückter spoke most warmly of Schulemann and the support and assistance he had provided throughout his career.[70] A fourth connection between Schulemann and thalidomide was also deep and personal. He

[67] Bonn University Year Book *(Jahrbuch)*, 1950, lists Schulemann as a member of the faculty since 1937 [sic – the formal appointment was in 1938], without any hint of his expulsion; Holldorf, August W., 'Schulemann, Werner', *Neue Deutsche Biographie* 23 (2007), S. 675-676 [Onlinefassung]; at: *http://www.deutsche-biographie.de/ppn117160164.html* <viewed 9 June 2015>.

[68] For example, phthalic acid / phthalimides in 1928 patent, US 1760781; CIOS report 24 XXIII-17 gives a picture of a glutarimide molecule similar to thalidomide on p. 15.

[69] Private communication with Dr. Harald Mückter, son of Heinrich Mückter, 8/9 December 2009.

[70] *Ibid.*

trained Dr. Herbert Keller, who, shortly after moving from Schulemann's institute at the University of Bonn to Chemie Grünenthal in 1954, became the co-inventor of thalidomide.[71] In his testimony at the trial of the Grünenthal staff in the 1960s, Keller, too, emphasised the close personal connection between Schulemann and Mückter:

> *In general, I cannot answer the question of who all advised us [Chemie Grünenthal] with concrete information – with the exception naturally of Professor Schulemann, with whom the top management, especially Dr. Mückter, had very lively contact. Prof. Schulemann had an extraordinary range of industrial experience. He had had top managerial posts with two important companies. He has a worldwide reputation as creator of AM [pharmaceuticals]. I presume that he always stood behind Dr. Mückter and monitored progress.*[72]

HEINRICH MÜCKTER (1914-1987)

The man Schulemann stood behind, Heinrich Mücker, and in particular Mücker's actions and affiliations during the Third Reich, formed the second node in the network that underpinned and enabled the thalidomide catastrophe. The development of his career starting in the 1930s demonstrates the way the connection emerged.

Immediately after completing his training as a medical doctor in 1940, Heinrich Mückter took up a posting at the Army Institute for Typhus and Virus Research (Institut für Fleckfieber- und Virusforschung des Oberkommandos des Heeres) in Kraków in the General Government (formerly part of Poland). He remained with the Institute for the duration of the war, even after it was forced to move to Bavaria between August 1944 and 19 January 1945 in the wake of the Red Army's invasion of the General Government.[73] For a newly qualified medical scientist, this posting offered great opportunities in the context

[71] Patent DE 1074584, 17 May 1954; Verfahren zur Herstellung von Derivaten von Amino-piperidin-2,6-dionen; inventors Dr. Keller, Dr. Kunz.

[72] Dagmar and Karl-Heinz Wenzel, *Der Contergan-Prozess* (Berlin: Verlag Wissenschaft und Forschung, 1969) Vol 2; pp. 64-65.

[73] CIOS Target Number 24/241; 'Institut für Fleckfieber- und Virusforschung des Oberkommandos des Heeres', by Joseph Smadel, Hans Schlumberger, and Eugene Soles, Medical Section, HQ ETOUS, 27-30 April and 16-17 May 1945. Dr. Heinrich Naeckten [sic] is listed as co-assistant leader of the Institut (p. 5), but this is clearly a transcription error, as is clear from the list of reports on p. 16 that indicate that they were co-authored by Heinrich Mückter.

of Nazi Germany, although again many of them proved not only unsavoury, but almost surely also criminal.

Mückter's boss at the Institute was its director, Professor Hermann Eyer, another protégé of Schulemann, and Eyer oversaw a variety of research and experimentation connected mostly with potential treatments and vaccines for typhus, but also involving other diseases. Eyer submitted an affidavit to the Nuremberg trials denying that this Institute had been connected with the typhus vaccine experiments on prisoners at Buchenwald,[74] despite being directly implicated by the diaries of Dr. Erwin Ding-Schuler,[75] who controlled the experiments in the camp but worked under the direction of a number of scientific organisations, including Eyer's Institute. By his own account in the affidavit, Eyer had visited Buchenwald in connection with his work, and it is well known that at least 150 prisoners died out of some 700 used for the typhus vaccine and remedy experiments in Buchenwald alone. Pharmaceutical tests took place at Auschwitz and other centres, and there is little doubt that Eyer and his staff, including Mückter, must have been involved in some of these because of their leading role in this work for the army.

At Buchenwald, in connection with typhus experiments, the Institute and its members came into contact with a range of other key organisations and people. As Eugen Kogon, a prisoner who survived the camp and who worked under Dr. Ding-Schuler, reported:

> *By the end of 1944 there had been twenty-four series of [typhus vaccine] experiments, the number of subjects in each ranging from four to forty and even sixty – on one occasion there were 145 in a group. The tests concerned the efficacy of typhus serums of different origin: the egg-yolk-sac culture produced by the Behring Works after the process worked out by Cox,*

[74] Hermann Eyer, 'Affidavit' (26 February 1947) in Document Book Handloser, Doc. No. 83, previously available at: *http://nuremberg.law.harvard.edu/php/pflip.php?caseid=HLSL_NMT01&docnum=636&numpages=2&startpage=1&title=Affidavit..&color_setting=C* <viewed 10 June 2015 >, but no longer available at this URL. Copy in possession of authors.

[75] Dr. Erwin Ding-Schuler, an SS doctor at Buchenwald who carried out experiments with typhus and yellow fever vaccines on concentration camp inmates, kept a diary which was heavily quoted in the published proceedings of the Nuremberg 'Medical Case' held in 1946/1947. He mentions a visit of Dr. Eyer from the Army Institute for Typhus and Virus Research in Krakow in his entry of 8 February 1943 and test vaccines manufactured at that Institute in entries of 10 January 1943 and July 1944. See Extracts from the Ding Diaries in Trials of War Criminals before the Nuremberg Military Tribunals under Control Council Law No 10, Vol. 1, Case 1: *The 'Medical Case': United States vs. Karl Brandt, et. al.* (Washington: USGPO, n.d. [ca. 1949]), pp. 563 and 562 and 571 respectively.

Gildermeister, and Haagen; the Weigl serum, produced from the entrails of lice by the Institute of Typhus and Vaccine Research of the Army High Command at Cracow [sic]; the Durand-Giroud serum, prepared from rabbit lungs at the Pasteur Institute, Paris; a dog-lung serum by the process developed by Cantacuzino, Bucharest and a Danish serum from mouse livers, both made available by Professor Gerhard Rose, chief of the Division for Tropical Medicine of the Robert Koch Institute, Berlin; certain drugs such as Nitro-Acridine and Methylene Blue from I G Farben (Professor Lautenschläger); Rutenol from the same firm...[76]

But what was Mückter's specific role in these activities of the Institute? The essential problem for the Institute's researchers, desperate to find effective and cheap vaccines against typhus, was that concentration camp prisoners were not suitable subjects because they were weak and starving. Instead, they needed people who were fit and healthy. Heinrich Mückter's solution was to recruit Polish civilians, who were told they were only needed to 'feed' the lice being used for vaccine production. By this means various drugs and vaccines could then be tested on them. The testimony of one Polish civilian describes her near-fatal illness arising from what she had believed to be an innocuous test during her work at Dr. Mückter's headquarters on Czysta Street, Kraków, and it is worth quoting at length:

Commission to Investigate Nazi Crimes
4 Mikolaja Street
Kraków

Over two years ago I came to Katowicki's branch of Commission to Investigate Nazi Crimes with an issue which I'm presenting to your attention. I was advised to give evidence in Kraków's branch because the occurrence had happened in Kraków in 1944 in the Typhus Institute (Czysta Street) / Institut für Fleckfieber und Virusforschung). Unfortunately, after visiting this institute I was very ill and I had a very serious surgical operation. The convalescence took a very long time, therefore I have decided to describe what happen to me on paper because I

[76] Kogon, E., *The Theory and Practice of Hell: the German Concentration Camps and the System Behind Them*, pp. 149-150.

believe that I was experimented upon. Anyway, in 1944 I had to find a job because my work card had expired. I got a message from Arbeitsamt that I will be sent to Germany as a labour worker. Obviously, I tried to avoid it. A friend of mine, who was working at the institute, helped me by hiring me as lice feeder. The group that I was assigned to was a new group. Shortly after adoption we found out that we would receive some injections, which were supposed to protect us from the trench fever, which symptoms are similar to malaria but it's caused by lice excreta in human blood. From the day of so-called inoculation we had to report with the detailed state of our health. Especially, what was interesting for the staff of the institute was the fact if we had a fever and how high was it. Other symptoms that we were asked about were headaches and ache of the shin-bone. These were symptoms typical for trench fever. Soon after, everybody was seriously ill. The illness of mine was very hard: in evening time a high fever – 41.3 Celsius. I remember it as the highest fever I've ever had. At the morning about 35 Celsius, this variation made me feel extremely exhausted. Apart from that, of course, headache and the worst ever ache of shin-bone. Shortly after, I wasn't able to come to the institute, and after few days I had a visitor. It was an armed soldier who was supposed to bring me to the institute. And we walked through the city from Dietla to Czysta Street (note: a distance of 2.5 kilometres). Our door-keeper – I remember, his name was Bertch, he was a priest or a monk – told me that because of my absence at the institute my paper will be sent to Arbeitsamt. On the other hand, he could see that I was totally exhausted, and I must admit, he wasn't the worst example of German. He asked me to wait and he went, probably to his boss and asked not to send me to Arbeitsamt but to move me to work at the laboratory, because apart from trench fever my legs were swollen, and as a result lice didn't like my blood. I must say, that this man at that time did me a great favour.

After I started my work at the laboratory I found out that the injection I received earlier wasn't an inoculation, but I was injected with very virulent germs of trench fever. I wasn't feeling very well for a long time, and other feeders in my group were ill as well. From what I found out ... few people were seriously harmed because the illness caused damage to their kidneys, and others were diagnosed with the meningitis. Eventually I got out of this and slowly got back to normality.

If you're interested in this case I can add that, from I heard, we were the first group experimented upon with these particular injections.

I am an owner of two identity cards from this institute and I can send you a photocopy of if or I can come to Kraków and present the originals.

Sincerely yours, [name withheld] [77]

It is worth underscoring that this testimony certainly does not appear to describe a situation where lice-feeders had been inadvertently cross-infected, but instead was the result of a failed experiment in relation to trying to find a cure for trench fever. And, although Mückter is not mentioned by name in the letter, it refers to work carried out at the institute where he worked. Moreover, other Polish testimony reinforces this more explicitly, describing Dr. Mückter as a brutal, arrogant doctor who had no compunction about beating and abusing prisoners.[78]

The truth was that the disastrous trench fever experiment formed only part of what might have been a criminal case against Mückter and Eyer had they not been protected from extradition by virtue of having moved into southwestern Germany towards the end of the war, which eventually meant they were on what was for them the right side of the Iron Curtain. The other part of the charge was a result of the nature of that flight from the General Government just before the arrival of the Red Army in Kraków: after the end of the war, Polish authorities prepared criminal charges against Mückter, and also Hermann Eyer, for forcing workers suffering from typhoid or long-term high fever (40°C+) to work, and also for the theft of the entire equipment of the Institute (including furniture and sanitary fittings) from Kraków University. The American army captured Mückter with the consignment of laboratory

[77] Information received from national Institute of National Remembrance, Warsaw, reference (Polish Ambassador, London) MBr 2837-01-07, copies in possession of authors.

[78] Steuer, Armin, 'Contergan-Erfinder kooperierte mit KZ', TAZ, 6 February1999 *http://www.taz.de/index.php?id=archivseite&dig=1999/02/06/a0047* <viewed 13 October 2015>.

equipment, but did not prosecute him. Instead, they returned the laboratory equipment to Kraków University.[79] Despite being caught red-handed with his looted goods, he never stood trial, although the charges remained valid in Poland. In later years, he told his son that he had a number of friends in Poland but was unable to visit them because he would have been arrested if he went there.[80]

Figure 6: Hazel Simmons with her mother Alexandria, 1965. Note the experimental (and dangerous) prosthetic legs fitted to this toddler.

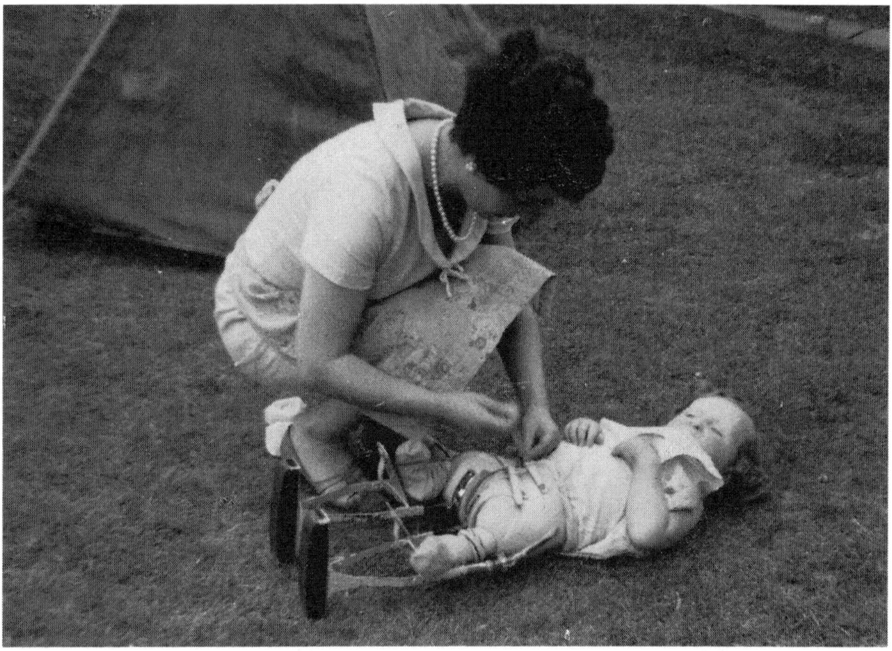

© Thalidomide Society on behalf of the copyright holder

DR. OTTO AMBROS (1901-1990)

The third person who formed a node in the personal, organisational and artefactual network that was constructed in the Third Reich and which underpinned and enabled the thalidomide disaster was Otto Ambros, a key member of the IG Farben managing board who was responsible, among other things, for the chemical firm's factory at Auschwitz and for its chemical and nerve warfare programme at

[79] *Ibid.*
[80] Interview with Dr. Harald Mückter, Munich, 8 July 2009.

Dyhernfurth.[81] The nature of Ambros's involvement in this network was different from the others in some respects: not only was he the only one of the three to face trial, conviction and imprisonment for his war crimes in conjunction with the use and maltreatment of slave labourers at the IG factory at Auschwitz (he was sentenced to eight years in prison, but was freed after just three years by the US High Commissioner in Germany, John McCloy); it is also unlikely that he met the other two face to face before the 1950s or, if he did so, it was almost certainly only Werner Schulemann.

Still, he deserves to be included here for three reasons. First, Ambros's prominence with IG Farben and his centrality in its crimes provide an important, if somewhat indirect, link to the crimes that have figured so prominently in this chapter. The story of IG Farben in the Third Reich has been told well and at great length,[82] but here it is worth highlighting Ambros's role in that story. He and others sought to create the most sophisticated integrated chemical production factory in the world at Auschwitz, and he pursued this dream of technological excellence. It remained a dream until the end because the factory never produced much of anything and certainly nothing of what it was supposed to manufacture in support of the war effort – regardless of the nightmarish consequences in human life and health. Even on the eve of his trial in Nuremberg, Ambros showed no remorse whatsoever, emphasising his pride in the potential technological achievement that IG Auschwitz represented.[83]

The second reason to include Ambros here is related to his close involvement in the chemical warfare programme. He headed up Anorgana GmbH, the IG subsidiary set up for this purpose at Dyhernfurth, and he is also recognised as a co-inventor of the nerve gas Sarin[84]. And although Tabun and Sarin were not deployed in combat during the war, they were particularly interesting to the Allied conquerors who entered Germany in 1945. What is particularly

[81] On Ambros and IG Auschwitz, see Raymond G. Stokes; 'From the IG Farben Fusion to the Establishment of BASF AG (1925-1952)'; pp. 206-361, passim, in Werner Abelshauser et. al., *German Industry and Global Enterprise: BASF: The History of a Company* (Cambridge/NY: Cambridge University Press, 2004); on Ambros and chemical warfare agents, see Jonathan B. Tucker, *War of Nerves: Chemical Warfare from WW1 to Al-Qaeda* (New York: Anchor Books, 2007) chapters 2 and 3.

[82] The key work here is Peter Hayes, *Industry and Ideology: IG Farben in the Nazi Era,* 2nd ed. (Cambridge/NY: Cambridge University Press, 2001).

[83] Stokes, 'From the IG Farben Fusion to the Establishment of BASF AG (1925-1952)', p. 343.

[84] The name SARIN was made from the initials of Schrader, Ambros, Rüdiger and LINde: Jonathan B. Tucker, *War of Nerves: Chemical Warfare from WW1 to Al-Qaeda,* p. 40.

important about all of this activity for our story is that there is a real possibility that thalidomide or a substance like it may have been invented during the war in connection with the nerve gas programme. And it is also worth noting that although Ambros was not charged in connection with his work on the nerve gas project, the fact remains that 3,000 Auschwitz prisoners who were drafted for testing to the nerve gas factory at Dyhernfurth died. Prisoners were also used as human 'canaries', locked up without gas masks in railway wagons or munitions depots where Tabun-filled (Tabun, like Sarin, was a nerve gas) munitions were being transported or stored.[85] Eugen Kogon has written that prisoners from many camps were used:

> *It took them only a few hours on each occasion, early in 1942, to compile lists of prisoners at Dachau, Sachsenhausen, Buchenwald, Mauthausen, Auschwitz, Flossenburg, Gross-Rosen, Neuengamme, and Niederhagen ... soon afterward the prisoners would be shipped to an unknown destination. A short time later – six hours to three days, depending on the location of the camp – the personal possessions of the prisoners, including the contents of their pockets and their dentures, would be returned to the camp. We soon learned that new poison gases had been tried on the prisoners. The gases had been previously tested on cattle. Among the very first to be shipped out of Buchenwald to be gassed in this way were a whole series of political prisoners, such as the Austrian security director from Salzburg, Dr. Bechinie. According to reports, the mental institution at Bernburg, near Köthen, was the scene of these special gassings.*[86]

Just to be clear: the only 'new poison gases' available in Germany at that time were the nerve agents Tabun and Sarin.

Finally, Ambros's inclusion here is important because he later had very close and direct connections to Chemie Grünenthal, some of which were the result of his activities before 1945. After all, under the terms associated with his early release from his prison sentence following his conviction in Nuremberg, there was an explicit commitment on his part to avoid direct involvement with the large successor firms to IG Farben

85 Jonathan B. Tucker, *War of Nerves: Chemical Warfare from WW1 to Al-Qaeda,* p. 51.

86 Kogon, E., *The Theory and Practice of Hell: the German Concentration Camps and the System Behind Them* (New York: Farrar, Strauss & Giroux, 1950) p. 218.

that were created by 1952.[87] Consequently, Ambros's subsequent career centred on consultancy, in particular in relation to non-German firms, and he also held directorships in small German companies. The former included W.R. Grace, the American chemical giant with which Ambros and IG Farben had a relationship before the Second World War, but also the Distillers Company, which purchased a licence for production and sale of thalidomide in the UK from Chemie Grünenthal in 1958.[88] The latter included a directorship of Knoll AG, a Ludwigshafen-based pharmaceuticals firm whose board in 1960 also included Hermann Wirtz, a member of the family that owned Chemie Grünenthal and whose membership of the board stemmed from a shareholding in Knoll purchased with the proceeds of the firm's thalidomide bonanza.[89] What is more, Ambros actually joined the Grünenthal board in February 1976.[90] In other words, Ambros, like Schulemann, formed a vital link between big and small chemical firms both in Germany and internationally.

The stories of these three men illustrate the combination of commercial, scientific, academic, political and technological networks which, taken together, made Grünenthal and the thalidomide disaster possible. The locations and organisations woven together within these networks included a number of notorious concentration camps, amongst which Auschwitz and Buchenwald are the most notorious; the University of Bonn; the world-famous Institut Pasteur in Paris; and the much less well-known and short-lived Army Institute for Typhus and Virus Research in Kraków. The chemical companies knitted together

[87] Otto Ambros, 'Memorandum', 14 November 1967, Ronald Reagan Library. From set of documents cited by Annie Jacobsen, *Operation Paperclip: The Secret Intelligence Program that Brought Nazi Scientists to America* (New York: Back Bay Books, 2014) p. 419. Copy of document in possession of authors.

[88] James W. Nance (White House) to Congressman Tom Lantos, 13 April 1982, Ronald Reagan Library, from set of documents cited by Annie Jacobsen, *Operation Paperclip,* p. 419. Copy of document in possession of authors.

[89] Otto Ambros to J. Peter Grace, Jr. (W.R. Grace & Co.), 30 January 1980, Ronald Reagan Library. Ambros noted in this document that when he was chairman of Knoll, the owners were the Arnsperger family (74.9 percent) and Chemie Grünenthal (25.1 percent). (From set of documents cited by Annie Jacobsen; *Operation Paperclip;* p. 419. Copy of document in possession of authors). See also: Thomas, U. (1986) *Knoll A.G., BASF-Gruppe. 100 Jahre im Dienste der Gesundheit: 1886-1986,* Knoll A.G., Ludwigshafen am Rhein (Germany), p. 158; Knoll A.G., *Geschäftsbericht 1960,* listing of members of Aufsichtsrat, including Ambros and Hermann Wirtz.

[90] Letter from Chemie Grünenthal Gmbh to the Amtgericht Eschweiler, Kaiserstrasse, 5180 Eschweiler, dated 29.04.1976, announcing the formation of the Aufsichsrat der Chemie Grünenthal Gmbh, with Dr. Otto Ambros named as one of three members from 09.02.1976. Copy held by Martin Johnson.

included Bayer, BASF and Schering in Germany, along with others in Germany and elsewhere. Not all of these organisations survived the war, of course, but even in those cases where the particular camp, institute or company did not last beyond 1945, the relationships among the people involved did. And here it is important that participation in and (at the very least) tacit acceptance of murder, enslavement and human experiments formed part of their shared CVs. In the pursuit of medical, scientific and technological excellence and commercial gain, these men and the many like-minded individuals around them demonstrated a complete disregard for normal human values, and attained what they eventually achieved only at the cost of wreaking havoc and extreme suffering. The disastrous consequences of this pattern of behaviour became evident in the thalidomide catastrophe, which featured the firm Chemie Grünenthal at its heart.

CHAPTER THREE

An Organisation for Disaster

Chemie Grünenthal GmbH and the construction of corporate DNA.

IT ALMOST READS LIKE THE PLOT of a piece of pulp fiction:

Within a few months of Germany's defeat at the hands of the Allies, in the midst of the rubble and under British military occupation, a family with a soap and perfume business that started in the mid-19th century decides to depart sharply from tradition by embarking on an entirely new business venture in the pharmaceuticals industry. The family hires as the start-up's chief scientific officer a young medic with some experience in drugs research and testing in Nazi-occupied Poland who is in the process of completing a one-year degree programme in pharmacology. He promptly returns the favour by rapidly developing and bringing to market an antibiotic, allowing the firm to turn a profit almost from the start.

Meanwhile, the chief scientific officer's research 'staff' – at first a single individual who is even less experienced and well qualified than the scientific officer himself – sets about developing new products. When in the early 1950s the start-up identifies sedatives as having excellent growth potential, that poorly qualified staff member, together with a recent graduate of the University of Bonn who has joined the company just weeks before, patents a new compound that fits the bill very nicely. The patent specification for it is remarkably detailed in its description of the drug's effects on human beings, this in spite of the fact that there has been little, if any, research on – and no testing of – this within the firm. Within three years – and just over a decade after the founding of the start-up – the new sedative is on the market, a huge and enormously profitable hit that attracts licensees from Britain, Sweden and Japan among others and that competes successfully with a rival product developed by CIBA, a well-established Swiss-based pharmaceutical and chemical firm with an excellent track record in research and development.

It may read like a plot summary of a bad novel, but at the same time it is the essence of the story that Chemie Grünenthal GmbH, the company responsible for the introduction of thalidomide, tells about itself for the years from its founding in 1946 until the late 1950s.[91] One virtue of recounting it in this highly compressed and stylised way is that it brings into sharp relief just how improbable the story is. The questions arise already with the first sentence:

- Why on earth did a family of soap and perfume manufacturers decide to go into the pharmaceuticals business?
- Where did they get the money to do so, especially in the context of the extremely limited resources available in defeated and occupied Germany in 1946?

And the questions cascade from that point in the story forward:

- How did a recently qualified pharmacologist come up with a marketable antibiotic at a time when many established firms with large research teams were having trouble doing the same?
- How did that pharmacist's even less qualified underling come up with a new and highly profitable sedative to order, and what was the role in this of the researcher who joined the company only weeks before the patent on this sedative was filed?
- How did the two of them know about the drug's effects even though they had done no testing when the patent was filed?

[91] See for instance quotations from the company in Armin Steuer, 'Contergan-Erfinder kooperierte mit KZ', *TAZ*, 6 February 1999: *http://www.taz.de/index.php?id=archivseite&dig=1999/02/06/a0047* <viewed 13 October 2015>; Chemie Grünenthal GmbH, 'The thalidomide tragedy' (offprint from 60th anniversary publication) (Stolberg: Chemie Grünenthal, 2007).

Finding definitive answers to these and other questions that arise from the story the company tells about itself is nigh on impossible. But we can highlight the issues at stake and make some plausible suggestions about the answers to these questions through a close examination of the story of Chemie Grünenthal from its establishment in 1946 into the 1960s. In particular, we focus on the networks and people we looked at in the last chapter as part of the explanation for the emergent corporate culture of the start-up.

The Wirtz family and the Dalli Group

The Wirtz family founded what would eventually become Dalli-Werke GmbH & Co. KG, or the Dalli Group, in Stolberg, near Aachen, in 1845, in order to make soap, and eventually also detergents and washing powder, businesses that, along with cosmetics, remain core activities of the firm to the present day. It also remains a family business, in its fifth generation. Into the 20th century, the firm grew and prospered, but remained relatively small, with about 150 employees on the eve of the First World War.[92]

It was, however, in particular during the Nazi period that the firm's fortunes soared. The reasons for that are not entirely clear, but there are some clues. Twins Hermann and Alfred Wirtz, born in 1896, and Artur, born in 1902, were the main protagonists here. The twins served in the Foot Artillery Regiment during the First World War, and were both awarded the Iron Cross.[93] They entered the family business after their return from military service. Artur joined the firm as well in the 1920s. He had been too young to join the army during the Great War, but he compensated for this later by joining the Nazi party; he was accepted for membership on 1 May 1933, not long after Hitler came to power. His brothers eventually decide that they wished to join the party as well but could not do so until later in the 1930s, mostly because the Party placed a moratorium on new memberships between 1 May 1933 and 1

[92] See information on the firm and its history available at: *http://www.dalli-group.com/* <viewed 3 August 2015>.

[93] Biographies of Wirtz brothers; report supplied to Jonathan Stone by Ruth Zeigler, 17 September 2007.

May 1937.[94] Artur, however, died in 1940, and his two brothers ran all the family businesses from then on. Hermann held the senior role in the Dalli group from 1930 until Grünenthal was founded. In 1946, he then took charge of newly formed Chemie Grünenthal until he retired, with Alfred subsequently in charge of Dalli. Hermann Wirtz was the director in charge of the family's new pharmaceutical operations for the whole of the period of the introduction of thalidomide, and then presided over the company's response to the catastrophe that followed.[95]

The Nazi period was not a good one for small soap-making firms. After all, as early as 1933 the regime began to limit the consumption of fat, the main ingredient for soap (and also margarine and various other products), with the aim of reducing this by half in order to save foreign exchange; an estimated 85% of Germany's fats were imported at the time. A number of plans were put in place to counter this problem, ranging from attempts to make synthetic fat out of coal to intensifying German whaling operations. In 1939, the government saw the situation as critical enough to create an agency specifically to control fat supply and regulate the soap industry. As a result of the controls and the limited success of plans to develop alternative supplies of fats, some soap and washing powder factories were forced to halt production; even the Henkel company had to suspend manufacture of their famous 'Persil' brand soap powder for a time. The most likely explanation for the fact that the Dalli group had a completely different experience during this period, not only surviving, but growing larger and prospering, is that its owners cultivated close contacts with the Nazi regime.[96]

There is additional evidence. In 1938, the number of employees in the Dalli Group ballooned to 700 through the acquisition of two substantial companies,[97] the Doering Werke in Berlin and Riva in

[94] Private correspondence between Stefan Krebs (author of *Zwangsarbeit in Stolberg/Rhld. Eine erstse Bestandsaufnahme* [Stolberg, 2003]) and Jonathan Stone, email 17 October 2007. Artur Wirtz's NSDAP membership is dated 1 May 1933, the last possible date to join the party before the moratorium, and Alfred and Hermann Wirtz joined on 1 October 1939. All three were 'simple' members of the local Stolberg branch (Ortsgruppe). They do not appear to have belonged to any other Nazi organisations (e.g. SA, SS etc.) Applications to join the Nazi Party were not accepted between 19 April 1933 and the late 1930s.

[95] Report for Martin Johnson by Inge Mecke, Corporate Research Clifford Chance CIS Ltd dated 22 February 2007.

[96] Report for Martin Johnson by Inge Mecke, Corporate Research Clifford Chance CIS Ltd dated 28 August 2007.

[97] See information on the firm and its history available at: *http://www.dalli-group.com/de/ueber-uns/historie.html* <viewed 3 August 2015>.

Vienna. Both had previously been largely Jewish-owned. As far as Riva Vienna is concerned, there is clear evidence that it was acquired for a fraction of its true market value as part of a process known as 'Aryanisation', and there is ground for suspicion that the same applies to the acquisition of Doering Werke. Companies that were Aryanised were thus in effect stolen from their owners in return for trivial sums of money that even then were not available to the 'beneficiaries' as they were paid to a blocked account. The Dalli Group faced legal challenges after the war in respect of the opportunistic takeover of Riva, but escaped any serious consequences other than the payment of modest compensation.[98] The Doering factory, based in what became East Berlin, was expropriated (without payment to the Dalli Group) by the Soviets. The Group therefore was not required to indemnify the previous owners in this case, but the simple fact that compensation had to be paid for Riva indicates that both of these acquisitions were highly problematic, indeed perhaps even criminal.[99]

During the war, the Dalli Group became a major supplier of soaps and detergents to the Wehrmacht,[100] providing goods that were especially important for hygiene in hospitals and other army medical facilities. As a favoured government supplier, the company thus enjoyed priority in the allocation of essential raw materials. The same was true with regard to supply of labour. During the war years, the main factory in Stolberg featured between 250 and 270 foreign – mostly forced and some slave – labourers, a number that probably approached half of the total work force of that facility. These people were mostly women from

98 Email from the director of the Vienna City Archive to Tobias Arndt, 26 February 2008 describes the Aryanisation of 'Riva' in Vienna, with the three Wirtz brothers named as party to the process, on 28 December 1938, and the presentation of claims for restitution lodged in 1956. Dalli group has managed to retain the 'Tabac' brand of men's toiletries that originated with Riva.

99 Doering Werke takeover by Wirtz family listed in Deutsche Wirtschaftarchive 1994 p. 54 eds. Klara van Eyll, Renate Schwärzel; Doering listed as a Jewish-owned business in Berlin at *http://www2.hu-berlin.de/djgb/www/find?sort=unternehmen&fq=Stadtbezirk%3A%22Wei%C3%9Fensee%22+AND+Branchen%3A%22Chemie+und+Drogeriewaren%22* published by Humboldt University Berlin, <viewed 6 August 2015> and this takeover also referenced in the company history: *http://www.dalli-group.com/de/ueber-uns/historie.html* <viewed 3 August 2015>.

100 'Dalli-Werke GmbH & Co. KG.', *International Directory of Company Histories* (2007): *http://www.encyclopedia.com/doc/1G2-2690200032.html* <viewed 5 August 2015>. 'During the war, under strict government administration and raw material restrictions, Maurer & Wirtz produced standardized soap and soap powders for the German army as well as new fat-free Dalli products for the German civilian population. The company's lab created additional new products using raw materials to which access was not restricted ... Production in Stolberg continued until the Autumn of 1944 when American Allied troops seized the region.'

Holland, France and Belgium who were compelled to leave their homes and go where German authorities directed, and they were eventually joined by a large number of Soviet prisoners-of-war (POWs) after the invasion of the Soviet Union in June 1941. Many of the women working in the soap factory had young children with them, and during their long shifts the children were left to fend for themselves in the workers' barracks. Food was in short supply, and those women workers who became pregnant were likely to lose their babies due to malnutrition, or, in the absence of adequate care, to die of the complications of childbirth.[101]

Although the Wirtz family was required to pay modest compensation for the opportunistic acquisition of the Jewish-owned factory in Vienna, and also in 1958 and 1959 for their use of forced and slave labourers in their main production facility, there were no other repercussions for their behaviour during the Nazi period. As a result, the family and their company entered the post-war period in very good financial shape and with a track record of corporate misbehaviour that, significantly, went almost entirely unpunished.

Figure 7: Amanda Kiddell, aged three months.

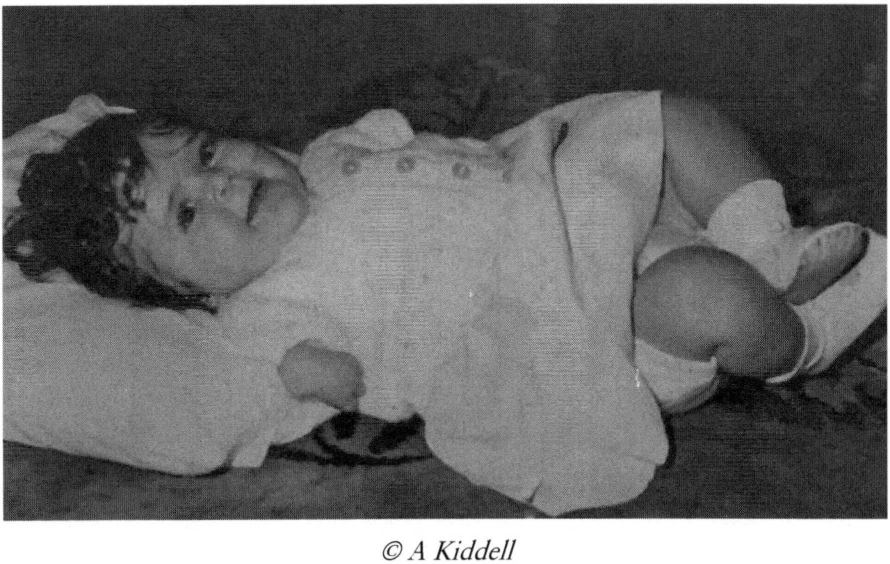

© A Kiddell

[101] Stefan Krebs, *Zwangsarbeit in Stolberg/Rhld. Eine ertse Bestandsaufnahme* (Stolberg, 2003), ISBN 3-926830-17-4, esp. pps. 157-159; also '...nach Auschwitz verzogen', Karen Lange-Rehberg, *Stolberg: Stationen von Nazi-Terror, Verfolgung und Widerstand im 'Dritten Reich'* (Stolberg: Gruppe Z, November 2011).

The establishment and early years of Chemie Grünenthal GmbH

The area around Aachen was one of the first parts of Germany to be occupied by Allied forces. Indeed, it was under Allied control already in late 1944, although the formal military occupation began only after the unconditional German surrender in May 1945. Aachen, Stolberg and the rest of the large and heavily populated state of North Rhine Westphalia became part of the British zone of occupation. Like much of the rest of defeated Germany and large swaths of other European countries where the fighting and bombing had occurred, it was a grim place in the second half of 1945 and for several years thereafter. But North Rhine Westphalia featured particular problems. The area was not only heavily populated; it was also heavily industrialised. But owing to destruction to factories and general economic collapse, there were few jobs. Limited income combined with severe inflation meant food could not be purchased in sufficient quantities, nor, in this highly industrialised and urbanised area, could adequate supplies be grown. Even though there was understandably little sympathy on the part of the Allied occupation authorities for the Germans, who had after all caused enormous destruction and loss of life during the war, it soon became obvious that they would have to provide extensive relief in order to fend off a humanitarian disaster that would involve widespread disease ac-companied by political unrest. The problem here was that Britain itself was in dire economic straits, and was therefore not in a position to provide that relief on its own. The result was a decision during 1946 to create an economic union with the American zone of occupation. The Bizone was duly created on 1 January 1947, which provided access to relief funds from the much wealthier American occupation authorities.

This is not the place to discuss the history of the occupation of Germany at any great length, but this short overview should make a key point abundantly clear: North Rhine Westphalia in late 1945 and early 1946 was not a promising business environment at all. Capital was in short supply, while consumers had little cash or other assets with which to purchase even basic necessities. On the other hand, there are business opportunities in any situation, in particular if capital is available for investment, and purveyors of soaps and detergents were in a potentially very good position because they supplied items crucial for helping prevent the disease and unrest feared by the occupiers. Producers of medicines were also in an excellent position for the same reason.

The Wirtz family, having prospered during the Nazi period, was certainly well placed in terms of capital for investment, and their core soap and detergent business had excellent prospects that were soon realised. Why exactly they decided to pursue a strategy of completely unrelated diversification into pharmaceuticals at this time is a bit of a mystery, although the very large growth potential here combined with what appear to have been close personal connections between the Wirtz family and Pharmacology Professor Werner Schulemann at the University of Bonn (whom we encountered for the first time in Chapter 2) may provide the explanation. The company's 'official' story is that their soap factory manager, Jakob Chauvistré, had some chance conversations with a pharmacist in an air raid shelter during bombing raids on Aachen which gave him the idea the firm should branch out into pharmaceuticals.[102]

This story is quite implausible, and we will return to the Schulemann connection shortly to try to suggest more plausible explanations for the decision to enter the new business. What is important just now is that, for whatever reasons, the Wirtz family decided sometime in late 1945 to go into pharmaceuticals. Chemie Grünenthal GmbH was duly registered as a company on 4 January 1946 with a share capital of 20,000 Reichsmarks (RM), which in 1946 approximated to US $2,000 at the official exchange rate.[103] It was a negligible sum to begin with, indeed the minimum amount legally necessary to register a new limited company at the time. By the end of the year, however, on 23 December 1946 to be precise, the shareholding was increased to RM 200,000 with money from the two Wirtz brothers.[104] Hermann Wirtz and Jakob Chauvistré, the Belgian

102 Grünenthal history, 1946-2006, *60 years of Grünenthal,* pub. Grünenthal GmbH, p. 6.

103 This equated to £500 UK: the official exchange rate 1946 £1=RM 40 but in reality such amounts in 'hard' currency could have bought many more Reichsmarks in those days. In January 1946 the Reichsmark was a 'busted' currency, with a negligible exchange rate, and potentially convertible into cigarettes, at the rate of about RM2 for one cigarette. (See Michael Howard; *Otherwise Occupied; letters home from the ruins of Nazi Germany* [Tiverton: Old St Publishing, 2010], pp. 70, 94 etc.) In 1948, at the creation of the Deutschmark, the decision to convert Reichsmarks to Deutschmarks came after three years of uncertainty: 1:1 for small cash allowance (60 DM). Savings a/cs converted at notionally 1:10, but in practice this dropped to 1:15. Bundesbank monthly report, March 2002, pp. 19-34 available at: *http://www.bundesbank.de/Redaktion/EN/Downloads/Publications/Monthly_Report_Articles/2002/2002_03_circulation_mark.pdf?__blob=publicationFile* <viewed 5 August 2015>.

104 RM 99,000 from Hermann Wirtz and RM 81,000 from Alfred Wirtz.

national who had been a key manager in the Dalli Group during the war and who allegedly had discussions about this business opportunity while bombs rained down on Aachen, became the registered directors on that date.[105]

Between the formal founding of the firm and this true 'launch date' in December of that year, however, there was another key milestone attained by the fledgling company. On 1 July 1946, Dr. Heinrich Mückter was appointed chief scientific officer on the personal recommendation of Professor Werner Schulemann, Mückter's teacher on his medical degree programme that he completed in 1940 and on the pharmacology programme that he was in the process of completing when appointed chief scientific officer. This would seem to make it clear that there was a close connection between this eminent scientist, who had and would continue to add large numbers of pharmaceutical patents under his name, and the Wirtz brothers.[106] This probable relationship offers the most plausible explanation for the brothers' decision to branch out into this completely new area of business.

Yet another – closely related – reason, though, was Mückter himself. We last encountered Dr. Mückter in Chapter 2 as a recently qualified medical doctor working in the Army Institute for Typhus and Virus Research in Kraków in German-occupied Poland during the war. There, he carried out research and testing of drugs on Polish civilians and possibly concentration camp inmates, and, in large part for this reason, he fled from there to Western Germany towards the end of the conflict. Formally discharged from the army in July 1945, Mückter soon started a one-year degree course in chemistry with a focus on pharmacology at the University of Bonn, where he had gained his medical qualification and where he had come to know Schulemann before the war. As he came towards the completion of his pharmacology qualification, Mückter later told his son he'd received two job offers, one from Schering AG at a very junior level, and one from newly formed Chemie Grünenthal. Schulemann had excellent

[105] Grünenthal company formation papers, dated 23 December 1946; Aachen commercial court archive.

[106] Contergan Trial Indictment dated 10 March 1967, p. 4: 'Durch die Vermittlung von Professor Dr. Schulemann kam Dr. Mückter am 1 Juli 1946 zur firma Chemie Grünenthal. Hier wurde er als Leiter der kosmetisch-pharmazeutischen Laboratorien, deren Herrichtung ihm übertragen wurde, eingestellt. Bereits damals vereinbarte die Chemie Grünenthal mit dem Angeschultigten eine "Umsatzvergütung für marketfähige Präparate, die aus dem kosmetisch-pharmazeutischen Laborbereich hervorgehen", -Mindesthöhe: 1% der Rechnungsbeträge.'

connections to both. Mückter decided to accept the second offer, which he believed would offer better long-term prospects.[107]

Less than three years after its founding, Chemie Grünenthal was flourishing as the first indigenous German manufacturer of a commercial antibiotic, apparently in no small part owing to the efforts of the company's chief scientist. The firm later gave an explanation of this extraordinary scientific (and commercial) achievement:

> *His [Mückter's career] path led him from field and forest preparations [i.e. natural remedies] almost as a matter of course to antibiotics. The experiences and insights acquired during his medical placement at the institute for typhus in Kraków led as a matter of course to experiments on mould with his new employer in Stolberg.*[108]

Let us stop here to make a key point: this story taxes credibility to the breaking point! Mückter's training, experience and qualifications at this stage in his career meant that he could probably be relied on to run a fairly run-of-the-mill pharmaceutical laboratory attached to a factory featuring small-scale production of established products. But the idea that he would come up with a penicillin-based antibiotic in his tiny and unsophisticated laboratory, assisted by Willi Kunz, a man with even less pharmaceutical background and experience than Mückter (and whom we will return to in more detail later),[109] and furthermore that this antibiotic would then be produced on a large scale in the still very new Grünenthal factory, does not ring true at all. The drive to create viable strains of penicillin, after all, was a major part of the scientific war effort on both sides of the Atlantic through 1945, with an extremely high priority, and that effort continued in the immediate post-war period. It was a highly sophisticated business because, while there are many common penicillin moulds, finding strains that could produce the required antibiotic in useable quantities was a very difficult task. Indeed, it was one which had defeated many of the top-rank scientists

[107] Dr. Harald Mückter interviewed by Martin Johnson, 8 July 2009, Munich.

[108] Quoted in Steuer, 'Der Contergan-Erfinder'.

[109] *The Sunday Times* Insight Team, *Suffer The Children: The Story of Thalidomide,* pp. 11-12.

working on it in sophisticated, well-equipped laboratories in large, highly qualified teams. This was particularly the case in Germany.[110]

That a young medical doctor recently qualified as a pharmacologist and his even less qualified and experienced assistant would have been able to outperform such experienced scientists practically is simply not believable. And, most importantly, despite extensive searches of the key patent registries, no trace has been found of any patent filed by Heinrich Mückter in respect of the penicillin which went into full production in 1948.

So where did the drug come from? We do not know for sure, but it seems very likely that the Grünenthal penicillin originated in the work of a French scientist, Charles Cosar, who worked at the Institut Pasteur in Paris and appears to have developed a close working relationship with Mückter during the war. The Institut Pasteur was closely involved in typhus vaccine development and testing of potential vaccines on inmates at the Buchenwald concentration camp, in close collaboration with Mückter's Institute in Kraków, as indicated by a number of diary entries by the chief organiser of the Buchenwald testing programme, Dr. Erwin Ding-Schuler.[111] Mückter in later years told his son of wartime visits to Paris, which almost certainly took place in connection with this work.[112] Given the interconnectedness of institutions, individuals and research focus, then, it seems very plausible that Mückter and Cosar formed a working relationship no later than 1944, when the latter was named as the inventor on a penicillin patent registered by the French pharmaceutical company, Rhône-Poulenc.[113] It is certainly a more likely explanation than the one put forward by the company. After all, this relationship with Cosar would have been one of the key things Mückter brought to the table when he was being considered for the post at Grünenthal in 1946, and it is likely that this was the source of the

110 Shama, G., 'Pilzkrieg: the German wartime quest for penicillin', *Microbiology Today* 30 (August 2003), pp. 120-123: '...The main industrial participants in German penicillin work were the constituent companies of IG Farben, Schering and Merck. These had all achieved notable success with synthesised compounds, but found the change in methodology difficult to make, despite the considerable fermentation experience that existed in Germany... The failure to bring together existing fermentation experience and the considerable fermentation capacity in Germany proved costly.'

111 In 'EXTRACT FROM THE AFFIDAVIT OF DR. ERWIN SCHULER, 20 JULY 1945, CONCERNING TYPHUS EXPERIMENTS', *Trials of War Criminals before the Nuernberg Military Tribunals,* Vol. 1, *The Medical Case* (Washington: US Government Printing Office, n.d. [c. 1949]), pp. 573, 564, 569.

112 Dr. Harald Mückter, interviewed by Monika Eisenberg and Martin Johnson; 9 December 2009.

113 Patents FR 913.991 dated 23 June 1944, FR 53,878 (addition to FR 913.991) dated 4 July 1944; both for methods of producing penicillin.

otherwise extremely improbable breakthrough to a commercial product not long after. The fact that Cosar was later registered as the inventor of a number of additional Grünenthal antibiotics patents in the mid-1950s[114] adds even greater plausibility to this alternative account of the development of the firm's first product.

That development, moreover, was not only likely to have been based on research done outside the firm by someone other than the chief scientific officer; it was also almost certainly done illegally. Penicillin was such a sensitive issue that in Western Germany the occupying powers, probably out of fear of competition for their own companies, banned German companies from research on, or production of, penicillin. Mückter ignored this ban and obtained the licence to experiment with penicillin in January 1948 by lying about the nature of this work.[115]

Regardless of any uncertainties surrounding this particular explanation for how Chemie Grünenthal came into possession of the means to produce antibiotics shortly after its founding, what is beyond any doubt whatsoever is that Mückter was a rainmaker for the new firm. Such was the success of its initial forays into penicillin production that by the end of 1948, the company's share value was recorded as 1.2 million deutschmarks (DM). This constituted a nominal growth of 600% on its initial capitalisation of RM 200,000 in December 1946, although the actual growth is actually understated here: the RM figure was in a debased currency, whereas the DM one was in the form of one of the most spectacularly successful currencies of all time. Grünenthal went on to expand its manufacturing of antibiotics in the late 1940s and early 1950s, an expansion that was commercially successful if sometimes medically and ethically suspect.

In the early 1950s, for instance, the company introduced a new antibiotic named Pulmo 500 (brand name in USA 'Neo-Penil'). This drug was first patented in Denmark in 1949,[116] by Leo Pharma, a Danish company which had already produced penicillin (during the

[114] Patents DE 1.002.336 dated 15 December 1954, DE 1.008.284 dated 30 March 1955, DE 1.041.038 dated 20 February 1957; all for streptomycin-based preparations.
[115] Steuer, 'Der Contergan-Erfinder'.
[116] Patent DK 74.087 dated 7 July 1949.

German occupation) in 1943,[117] and from whom Grünenthal presumably obtained a licence. In 1954 and again in 1956, researchers published critical reports of this drug, the side effects of which included serious allergic reactions and even several fatalities, at a rate about 130 times greater than normal (procaine) penicillin. A very critical article in 1956 by three West German scientists, Wichmann, Koch and Hess, reported that the product had been 'used in man before thorough experiments on animals had been published', which they noted was certainly contrary to the ethics of more reputable firms.[118] Mückter and Grünenthal took no action to inform the medical profession about the side effects or to withdraw it, and in fact, surprisingly, the company escaped being taken to task over this dangerous product.[119] It was a pattern of behaviour that conformed uncomfortably to what had occurred in connection with Mückter during the war, while the cavalier approach to testing a new product combined with resistance to calls for it to be withdrawn once problems were identified seem very similar to the company's approach to thalidomide a few years later.

Patenting thalidomide and bringing it to market

The impressive financial success of Grünenthal's early penicillin production lasted barely five years. By the early 1950s, major American and British companies were producing antibiotics in larger quantities, at much lower prices and with much higher quality than Grünenthal could compete with. The company records show that by 1954 they made a profit of just DM 630,000 on a turnover of DM 21 million – a worrying situation to say the least. A 'profit and loss' transfer contract between Grünenthal GmbH and Dalli Werke Maurer & Wirtz KG in 1955 indicates funds being transferred into Grünenthal in exchange for

[117] This claim is made in Leo Pharma's company history available at: *http://www.leo-pharma.com/41256A84002BE7FC/adbdi/05CD38C3489EBAB3C1256AB50037E9AA?OpenDocument* <viewed 3 February 2010>. The company history indicates that the scientist who developed the penicillin 'managed to elude the German occupational forces that were heavily interested in obtaining penicillin.'

[118] Wichmann, Koch and Heiss, *Zeitschrift fur Klinische Medizin* (1956). As Sjöström and Nilsson point out (*Thalidomide and the power of the drug companies,* p.35) about the article, 'They particularly pointed out that "the penicillin ester was used in man before thorough tests on animals had been published". Although testing on animals at that time was certainly done on a more modest scale than now, clinical use in man before exhaustive tests had been conducted on animals was certainly against the ethics of more reputable firms.'

[119] Henning Sjöström, Robert Nilsson, *Thalidomide and the power of the drug companies,* pp. 33-35.

a part of Hermann Wirtz's shareholding.[120] Grünenthal was therefore being propped up by its sister company, Dalli, at this vulnerable point in its early years.

Clearly, something needed to be done to reverse the trend towards lower profitability and even losses. The identification of a new strategy for the firm was not long in coming, and it was followed remarkably quickly by a spectacular reversal of the trend in the firm's financial performance. As one former Grünenthal employee, Karl-Heinz Enderes, who joined the firm as an apprentice in 1954, remembered in 2007, a market analysis produced not long before his arrival at the company showed that there was a market for a non-toxic hypnotic sedative:

> *Dr. [Willi] Kunz was commissioned with the development of a compound and found it. The preparation [i.e. thalidomide] was on the market within three years. It all happened very quickly.*[121]

And, we might add yet again, it all happened quite implausibly, at least in the official company version of events. We will go into the many issues raised by the patent specification in Chapter 4, but it is worth stressing here again that 'Dr. Kunz' was the very same Willi Kunz who allegedly assisted Heinrich Mückter in the development of Grünenthal's initial successful antibiotic by 1948. Kunz was, however, a man with exceptionally limited qualifications and which were quite at odds with his elevated position in the firm and alleged accomplishments. In his war service, by 1945, he only reached the rank of sergeant (implying no education beyond basic high school), but he somehow obtained a PhD between 1945 and the end of 1953 while at the same time working during almost all of this period full-time for Grünenthal![122] It is implausible that a man with such a limited education and dubious doctoral credentials should have been capable of co-inventing viable pharmaceutical products, as indicated in the original patent specification for thalidomide.

120 Grünenthal company records for 1954 and 1955 in Aachen commercial court archive: a clerk's note on the fees for the company register in 1954 records annual profit DM 630,000, turnover DM 21 million. The 1955 'profit and loss transfer contract between Grünenthal GmbH and Dalli-Werke Mäurer & Wirtz KG' show that Hermann Wirtz lost voting shares as a result.

121 Michael Lehnberg, 'Der Augustiner Karl-Heinz Enderes hat die Entwicklung von Contergan hautnah mitverfolgt. Kleine Pille mit fatalen Folgen', *General Anzeiger Bonn,* 7 November 2007, available at: *http://www.general-anzeiger-bonn.de/index.php?k=loka&itemid=10001&detailid=376697* <viewed 4 May 2009>.

122 *The Sunday Times* Insight Team, *Suffer The Children: The Story of Thalidomide,* pp. 11-12.

There was, however, a co-inventor of the new compound listed on the initial patent for thalidomide from 1954 who was considerably better qualified than Kunz, but here, too, there is some significant improbability to what allegedly happened. There is no doubt about the basic fact that Dr. Herbert Keller joined the firm in February 1954, fresh from the University of Bonn where he had worked – unsurprisingly, perhaps, given the material we presented in Chapter 2 – with Professor Werner Schulemann. Just three months after Keller joined the company, moreover, the first patent for what was soon to become the company's flagship drug, thalidomide, was filed. By 1955, company employees were already sending out samples of the drug for 'clinical testing'.[123] The drug was then introduced commercially in Germany and most of Western Europe, along with Canada, Japan, the UK and Australia among other countries, between 1956 and 1958. It was a spectacular commercial success, competing successfully with such products as Doriden, a flagship sedative of the distinguished Swiss pharmaceutical company CIBA.[124] Not incidentally, thalidomide also helped boost the *earnings* of Chemie Grünenthal to over DM 69 million in 1960, more than triple the company's *turnover* just five years earlier. Sales of Contergan (the brand name used in Grünenthal's domestic market) in Germany alone soared from only DM 300,000 in 1958 to nearly DM 10 million in 1960, and were accelerating through 1961, reaching nearly DM 1.4 million a month in both March and May 1961, before a sharp fall-off to below DM 600,000 in September that year. The drug was withdrawn from the market at the end of November, with predictable effects on sales and earnings. When sales of other brand names and in other countries are included, it is clear that

[123] Letter from Dr. Piacenza to Dr. Mückter, dated 25 March 1956, indicating that Piacenza was disappointed with the results of his testing with K17 (Contergan). The medication had not lived up to its non-toxic billing and in fact had caused a range of side effects and there was 'absolute intolerability' in some patients and the drug had caused paraesthesia in one patient. This case was recorded following treatment with the drug on 25 November 1955, with a total of three 25mg tablets. Dr. Mückter's reply dated 3 April 1956 says 'we have been testing K17 [the company's internal designation for thalidomide' in many clinics and various sanatoriums for about 2 years, but had never received a negative report. Summary of and extracts from document in 'Affidavit of Michael Magazanik as to the Plaintiffs Case against the First Defendant (Grünenthal GmbH) Supreme Court of Victoria at Melbourne SCI 2011 3527,' 13 July 2012, pp. 18-20.

[124] Nils Kessel, '"Doriden von Ciba": sleeping pills, pharmaceutical marketing, and Thalidomide, 1955-1963', *History and Technology* 29 (2013): 153-168.

thalidomide was responsible for at least one third of total company turnover in 1960 and 1961.[125]

In other words, 'it all happened very quickly'[126] indeed! But did it happen the way the firm and its employees have repeatedly said it did? To answer that question, we need to look critically and in detail at the way the drug was patented and marketed, focusing initially on yet another question, one which was posed by Dr. C.G.H. Newman in 2008,[127] and which formed the impetus for the research for this book: *How did they know* what was published in the patent specification?

[125] Chemie Grünenthal GmbH balance sheet for the 1960 financial year; Aachen Commercial court archive; Contergan German sales 1958 (est) DM 300,000; 1959 (est) DM 2,000,000; 1960 DM 9,778,765; 1961 DM 11,778,674: Beate Kirk, *Der Contergan Fall* (Stuttgart, 1999) p. 57.

[126] Michael Lehnberg, 'Der Augustiner Karl-Heinz Enderes hat die Entwicklung von Contergan hautnah mitverfolgt. Kleine Pille mit fatalen Folgen', *General Anzeiger Bonn,* 7 November 2007, available at: *http://www.general-anzeiger-bonn.de/index.php?k=loka&itemid=10001&detailid=376697* <viewed 4 May 2009>.

[127] Dr. C.G.H. Newman at a meeting of the Thalidomide Trust in Leeds, on 9 October 2008 when he first saw the English version of the original Grünenthal patent for Thalidomide. See Chapter 4 for further details.

CHAPTER FOUR

Mechanism for Mayhem

Finding and patenting thalidomide.

Introduction

SO HOW *DID* THE 'INVENTORS' of thalidomide at Chemie Grünenthal discover what they wrote in their official patent specification? The answer to that question is not straightforward at all, and it must often be speculative. But, not surprisingly, given the material we presented in the two previous chapters, it revolves not only around the networks of people and organisations established in the National Socialist period, but also around the emerging corporate culture of Chemie Grünenthal.

To start with, we need to explain why it was that Dr. Claus Newman asked his deceptively simple question – 'How did they know that?' – at a meeting of the Thalidomide Trust in Leeds in 2008 after he had read the patent specification for the first time.[128] To do that, we must establish what the scientists and managers at Chemie Grünenthal seemed to know based on that patent specification, and why it was quite so odd that they apparently knew it. From there, we need to explore Dr. Newman's question more directly and thoroughly, examining various plausible – if ultimately also unprovable – scenarios.

[128] Dr. C.G.H. Newman at a meeting of the Thalidomide Trust in Leeds, on 9 October 2008 when he first saw the English version of the original Grünenthal patent for Thalidomide.

What they seemed to know and why it was so odd that they appeared to know it

Chemie Grünenthal filed the first of several patents for thalidomide-type compounds in West Germany on 17 May 1954, which eventually covered five different products, only one of which is now known as thalidomide. Within a year, patents were registered in neighbouring European countries and the USA, and subsequently in many other countries around the world. The first British patent for the new drug, filed on 29 April 1955, and the identically worded US patent from 16 May of the same year described the effects of thalidomide as follows:

> *The products of the invention possess valuable therapeutic properties. They cause a strongly pronounced lowering of the motility, i.e. the phenomenon of motion, and have a very low toxicity. They may be generally employed for 'central attenuation' (vegetative dystonia). The products of the invention do not have any peripherally paralysing curare-like effects.*
>
> *In addition, the compounds have certain spasmolytic and antihistaminic effects. Dispensed in larger quantities, the products of the invention, and particularly 3-phthalimido-2,6-dioxopiperidine [i.e. pure thalidomide] are effective as soporifics...*[129]

In other words, Drs. Herbert Keller and Willi Kunz, the inventors named on the first and on many of the other patents, appeared to know quite a lot, especially about the effects of the drug on the human body. Just how much they knew requires just a bit more unpacking. The most important point here is that the first set of patents described five extremely specific effects on the nervous system, which need some explanation, not least since the translation from the original German patent used in the English and American patents uses terms uncommon in English. The five effects were these:

- *'...strongly pronounced lowering of the motility...'*
  Here, 'motility' is being used to translate the German word 'Motilität', which relates to movements controlled by the autonomic nervous system. In English, in contrast, the word motility is generally used to refer to gastrointestinal motility

[129] UK 768821; USA 2830991.

(which might have been a reason for promoting the drug as a remedy for morning sickness). The word 'motility' as used here may well have involved both meanings, thus probably implying that the drug may affect the heart, circulatory and digestive systems.

- *'...central attenuation (vegetative dystonia)...'*
  The word translated as 'vegetative' refers in its German original to the autonomic nervous system, while 'Dystonie' (the original German word) means a disturbance in nerve transmission. The whole expression intends to show that the product interferes with the autonomic nervous system. There is not a directly comparable English term, though the French patent filed by Grünenthal uses the translation 'la dystonie neuro-végétative'[130] which confirms that this description is for a range of possible effects on the autonomic nervous system.
- *'...not peripherally paralysing (curare-like)...'*
  Curare's chief property is that it paralyses the main skeletal muscles, and also those used for breathing, but does not affect the heart muscles. It acts by antagonising acetylcholine, and it should be noted that this is not a mechanism normally associated with anticonvulsants.
- *'...spasmolytic ... effects.'*
  Here, the patent indicates that the drug acts as an anti-convulsant, stopping muscle spasms.
- *'...anti-histaminic effects.'*
  This statement indicates that thalidomide was claimed to oppose the action of histamine.

This is all a bit technical, but the key point is that these five separate descriptions demonstrate clearly that the writers of the patent apparently knew in great detail that the substances being described were expected to act on the autonomic nervous system of people in such a way that it caused the slowing down of muscle movements (without causing paralysis) and created a sedating or tranquilising effect. The overall effects would probably result in muscle relaxation and also affect organs controlled by the parasympathetic nervous system (digestive tract, heart, circulatory system).

[130] French Patent no. L164.512, registered 17 May 1955 in Paris.

But why is it so odd that the scientists appeared to know these details? Shouldn't they have? Here, we have to rehearse some of the details of the implausible creation myth promulgated by Chemie Grünenthal – which is also, and quite uncritically, generally accepted in scholarly literature and among the general public – setting them alongside the well documented and extremely poor scientific practice of the firm and its employees.

The story's implausibility arises in the first instance from claims about timing which have been made by Chemie Grünenthal and are broadly accepted. Briefly, the key facts are these: Dr. Herbert Keller joined the chemical firm in February 1954 from the University of Bonn, mainly to help develop a new sedative for the company, an area it had not long before identified as having real market potential. Just three months after Keller became an employee of the company, he and Dr. Willi Kunz, a member of the firm's research staff since its inception in 1946 who had extremely dubious qualifications, filed the first patent for what was soon to become the company's flagship drug, thalidomide. By 1955, samples of the drug were already being sent out for 'clinical testing'. The drug was then introduced commercially in Germany and most of Western Europe between 1956 and 1958.

This is an extremely compressed timeframe within which to introduce a new drug, even one which had potentially high demand at the time as a possible substitute for barbiturates, and which had attractive qualities (but also likely significant and dangerous side effects). Here, the 'career' of Librium demonstrates important parallels to that of thalidomide, but also a significant contrast. It, too, was developed in a search for a hypnotic sedative (just as was claimed for thalidomide) with the aim of replacing barbiturates. What is striking in contrast to thalidomide, though, is the length of time it took to come to market. Initial research by Dr. Leo Sternbach of Hoffman LaRoche began already in the 1930s, when he was a postdoctoral fellow. In 1954, he revisited his pre-war work and after some 18 months synthesised the compound that is now branded as Librium. In 1957, he put it forward for clinical evaluation, but it was only in 1960 the drug received Food and Drug Administration (FDA) approval.[131] In other words, from initial research work to approval took well over two, and nearly three, decades for Librium. In contrast, the creation myth for

[131] *http://www.benzo.org.uk/librium.htm* <viewed 27 November 2014>.

thalidomide posits a time frame of about two to three years between initial research and the drug being placed on the market. Thalidomide really *did* appear on the market with astonishing rapidity after its initial discovery even by the casual regulatory standards prevailing at the time.

But if the rapidity with which the drug was first discovered and then brought to market is so startling as to be unbelievable, especially given the detail provided in the patent specification, the testing regime which the firm allegedly undertook for the drug – which is well documented – renders the story completely implausible because it is entirely at odds with the depth of knowledge indicated in the patent specifications or in subsequent claims about the 'safety' of thalidomide used in selling the drug once it came onto the market.

Grünenthal filed a considerable number of patents in respect of thalidomide, beginning in West Germany. The first set of five was filed between May 1954 and May 1955 (see Appendix 1). Each of them was made on behalf of Chemie Grünenthal GmbH, and most identify the inventors as Drs. Keller and Kunz. These very first patents for thalidomide-like substances in turn list seven different processes, only one of which (the fifth) produces thalidomide as it was eventually marketed. Of the other processes, five are for thalidomide derivatives, with an extra chemical group added (Ethyl thalidomide, Methyl thalidomide and Allyl thalidomide), and one (the second process) is for a different compound completely. Testing, however, was only mentioned for the compound produced by the first process (Ethyl thalidomide), and only for mice. What is more, the claim here was that the 'LD 50' figure (Lethal Dose 50% – the amount of the compound that will kill half of the treated animals) was higher than 120 milligrams for each 20 grams body weight of mouse. This translates to six grams of drug for every kilogram of body weight – an enormous dose. They also claimed that mice are sedated at 10 milligrams of drug for each 20 grams body weight of mouse, or half a gram per kilogram. But it is important to underscore that these effects were claimed for *Ethyl* thalidomide, a different and derivative compound from pure thalidomide. The full significance of this will become clear shortly.

For now, it is worth noting that the next four patents, all filed in 1955 in the UK, Switzerland, the USA and France each reference the first German patent, but add a further seven manufacturing processes to the list, including six more ways of making thalidomide as it was eventually sold. Even so, the only test information given was that for the first process listed (the derivative Ethyl thalidomide). In other words, the intervening twelve months involved the firm identifying six more processes for making thalidomide without carrying out any further safety tests.

To reiterate, the initial patents only mention test results for mice, and a 1956 paper by Kunz et. al. described how the Grünenthal staff carried these out. The test method was very primitive and involved dosing the mice with thalidomide, placing them in a wire 'jiggle' cage and then suspending them over a sulphuric acid bath to see how much they moved about. If they did, electrodes beneath the cage dipped into the sulphuric acid and completed an electrolytic circuit, causing the acid to release hydrogen, which was captured at the top of the apparatus and measured. The measurements were then used as an indicator of the rate of mouse activity, although they would only have been able to indicate the crude amount of movement by the treated mice. The tests could not indicate even something as simple as whether the mice were actually asleep or not, let alone any physiological effects of the drug.[132] Here, it is crucial to note that no other pharmaceutical company ever appears to have relied on such rudimentary methods to determine the general effects or 'safety' of a drug.[133] The key point, though, is this: there is no conceivable way that the detailed information about the range of effects of the compounds given in these five patents can have been derived from the jiggle cage tests, and there are no contemporary records of any other tests which would have revealed this information.

What allegedly followed after this initial testing using jiggle cages was a wide range of tests on other animals. The same 1956 paper that reported the jiggle tests also noted the testing, in addition to 50 mice, of one dog, 20 rats, 20 guinea pigs and 10 rabbits. The report's only findings were that there was a lack of any obvious toxicity caused by the drug, again on the basis of some fairly rudimentary criteria.[134]

What is more, it is far from clear precisely what compound the tests reported in this paper involved! After all, Grünenthal referred to all nine or so products of its patents as compound K17. When Dr. Keller

132 The Grünenthal tests are reported in: Kunz, W., Keller., H., and Mückter, H., 'N-Phthalyl glutaminsaure-imid. Experimentelle Untersuchungen an einem neuen synthetischen Produkt mit sedativen Eigenschaften.', *Arzneimittelforschung* 6, 8: 426-430.

133 *The Sunday Times* Insight Team, *Suffer The Children: The Story of Thalidomide,* pp. 16-19.

134 Kunz, W., Keller., H., and Mückter, H., 'N-Phthalyl glutaminsaure-imid experimentelle Untersuchungen an einem neuen synthetischen Produkt mit Sedativen Eigenschaften', *Arzneimittelforschung* 6, 8; 426-430.

and Dr. Kunz were asked separately during the trial whether the version of K17 actually marketed as Contergan was the one they had tested, each answered that they did not know.[135]

But this is not the only puzzling aspect of the story. Indeed, a central mystery in the thalidomide disaster lies in the fact that Grünenthal claimed that all the records of the test results for thalidomide had been lost. Heinrich Mückter, Keller (by then a professor) and others gave evidence that they had conducted a wide range of tests on animals but, astonishingly, Mückter claimed in his testimony that all these records had disappeared during a move of premises.[136] One further complication of this puzzle appeared in an internal Distillers (the UK licensee of the drug) memorandum dated 15 December 1959 which was written by Dr. D.P. Young to N.F. Baker and three other colleagues at the company. In it, Young described attempting to replicate the processes specified in the original Grünenthal UK patent 768,821, but indicated that 'in most cases we get results other than those claimed'. In fact, in only 1 out of 14 trials was his team able to replicate the Grünenthal results, and several of the processes even resulted in the production of completely different chemicals from those specified in the patent. He concluded, 'I fear that it might be difficult to uphold this patent if a competing firm challenged its workability.' As the patent only protected the manufacturing processes, and not the end product, this was as good as saying the patent was useless.[137]

To sum up, then: we have a set of patent specifications which are far too detailed in their description of effects on humans given that, first, the testing regime that was undertaken *after* the patent was filed, and second, descriptions of the tests were very vague in terms of product and process. The former is the greater mystery, which we need to address directly and fully in due course; the latter, however, will eventually provide us with some clues about how to solve it.

[135] Dagmar and Karl-Heinz Wenzel, *Der Contergan-Prozess* vol. 2, p. 58 (for Wenzel and Wenzel summary of Keller testimony) and p. 74 (for Kunz testimony).
[136] Henning Sjöström, Robert Nilsson, *Thalidomide and the power of the drug companies,* pp. 188-189, 231-232.
[137] LAV NRW R, Gerichte Rep 139 Nr. 167c, Memo by Dr. Young dated 15 December 1959 (receipt stamped 17 December 1959).

How, then, did Chemie Grünenthal apparently know what was specified in the patents?

The short answer to the question posed in the heading of this subsection of the chapter is: in spite of years of research to try to get to the bottom of just this issue, *we just don't know for sure!* But our research allows us to put forward some plausible scenarios, all of which revolve around the strong likelihood that thalidomide was developed outside of Chemie Grünenthal; if so, quite probably also before 1954. It is even possible that it was developed during the Nazi period, and we will provide circumstantial evidence that lends some credence to this hypothesis, although there is also another possible explanation based on the vagueness of the product and processes in the patents for how the patentees knew so much about the effects of thalidomide on humans without allegedly having done any testing on human beings.

Telling this part of our story is not only controversial at times; it is also occasionally convoluted because the plot lines sometimes overlap, often in suggestive and intriguing ways. We will tell it as clearly as we possibly can.

Let's start by making the important point that we are not the first to suggest that thalidomide originated outside of Chemie Grünenthal. Indeed, in a report commissioned by US military authorities in Germany to explain why American army personnel serving there did not appear to have been affected by the 'German Outbreak of Phocomelia' between the late 1950s and 1961, Dr. Helen Taussig commented that:

> *Thalidomide is a synthetic drug which, as the story is told in West Germany, was first conceived and made by CIBA and found by them to have no effect on animals; therefore it was discarded.*[138]

We also can bring this line of inquiry in the discussion to a quick end by stressing that Taussig's claim was almost certainly not true. No records have been found evidencing any connection between CIBA and thalidomide, and independent research into the question has shown this was clearly not the case, and that there has been confusion between

[138] Taussig, Helen B., 'A Study of the German Outbreak of Phocomelia; the Thalidomide Syndrome', *The Journal of the American Medical Association* (June 30, 1962) Vol. 180; pp. 1006-1114.

thalidomide and Doriden, a CIBA sedative that competed with thalidomide.[139]

But the general point lurking behind Taussig's suggestion is significant: large pharmaceutical companies undertake research that results in the synthesis of a huge number of compounds, most of which are not pursued further by the large firm in question, but some of which might be picked up by smaller ones for development. Here there is a clear candidate in relation to thalidomide: the French firm Rhône-Poulenc.

Why? There are several reasons. First of all, Rhône-Poulenc worked closely with various IG Farben pharmaceutical divisions and the Institut Pasteur in Paris during the Nazi period to develop typhus drugs and vaccines that were tested on inmates at Buchenwald and other concentration camps – work that, as we have seen in Chapter 2, Dr. Heinrich Mückter had been closely involved in during the war years. So, there were established personal and professional connections there (as well as a proven willingness to carry out medical experiments on unwilling and/or uninformed human subjects). What is more, these relationships continued after the war. For instance, Grünenthal's own company history, published to mark its 60th anniversary in 2006, noted that the firm concluded a licence agreement with Rhône-Poulenc for streptomycin in 1951.[140]

But there is, of course, more. During the 1940s, Rhône-Poulenc registered at least 14 drug brand names, all ending with '(e)rgan',[141] among which was Antergan, which was tested in 1943 by Professor Richard Kuhn as a possible nerve gas antidote. Contergan, the brand name used for thalidomide in Germany (and, like Antergan, deriving from ancient Greek words with very similar meanings which can be translated as 'work against', or the more familiar Latin-derived word

[139] Yonkman, Frederick F., 'Thalidomide and related Compounds', *The Journal of the American Medical Association* (August 18, 1962) Vol. 181 (7): 654. Nils Kessel, '"Doriden von Ciba": sleeping pills, pharmaceutical marketing, and Thalidomide, 1955-1963', *History and Technology* 29 (2013): 153-168.

[140] *Der eigene Weg,* company publication 2007. Rhône Poulenc 1951 licence agreement p. 11.

[141] These included Antergan (1942), Salvhyrgan (1942), Antallergan (1943), Doxergan, Neo-Antergan (1945), Pamergan, and Phenergan (1947), Fenergan (1948), Lisergan (1950), Multergan (1951). Antergan, Antallergan, Neo-Antergan, Lisergan and Phenergan were drugs affecting the nervous system synthesised by scientists of Rhône-Poulenc working in conjunction with the Institut Pasteur in Paris under the supervision of Daniel Bovet: Winter, C. A., *A Study of Comparative Anti-histaminic Activity of Six Compounds* (Rahway, NJ: Merck Institute for Therapeutic Research, 1947); Bovet, D., 'Introduction to antihistamine agents and Antergan derivatives', *Annals of the New York Academy of Sciences* 9 (28 April 1950): 1089-1126.

'antidote'), was not one of those registered in the early 1940s, but it was eventually owned by Rhône-Poulenc. Indeed, the French company actually licensed the name to Chemie Grünenthal for exclusive use in Germany as indicated in a 6 August 1958 letter from Astra International to its Norwegian subsidiary, Norsk Astra, which was introduced as evidence during Astra's trial in Sweden in the 1960s. (Astra had purchased a licence from Grünenthal to allow it to produce and sell thalidomide in Scandinavia.) The letter ('to be treated as strictly confidential') pointed out that Astra 'cannot use the name Contergan in the Scandinavian countries, since Grünenthal obtained the name exclusively for the German market through an agreement with Rhône-Poulenc'.[142] This is not an isolated piece of evidence for this fact. In response to a query about the origins of thalidomide, representatives of the Hoechst division of Sanofi Aventis (the company formed through a merger of Hoechst, Rhône-Poulenc and other pharmaceutical firms) confirmed in March 2011 that Contergan was originally a Rhône-Poulenc trademark, but said that Rhône-Poulenc 'had never marketed thalidomide under that name'.[143]

But what does all of this mean? It is of course possible that the licence Rhône-Poulenc sold to Grünenthal only involved the use of the brand name, Contergan, and not, additionally, the rights to the manufacture and sale of thalidomide itself, which would mark the end of this line of inquiry. On the other hand, however, that would seem to be commercial nonsense. After all, Grünenthal staff had no difficulty in inventing brand names for the products they introduced prior to thalidomide. When they started marketing that drug, moreover, they and their licensees went on to invent or authorise at least another 48 names for it. In fact, thalidomide was first test-marketed under the trade name Grippex a year before it was introduced as Contergan. Very shortly thereafter, distribution of the drug outside of Germany took place under the Softenon trademark. In other words, the company clearly had no need to pay good money to purchase the trade name Contergan if thalidomide had been invented there in the first place. This suggests that acquisition of the rights to the trade name may have been connected to the acquisition of the rights to manufacture and distribute

142 Astra International to Norsk Astra A.S., 6 August 1958. Original letter held by Föreningen för de Neurosedynskadade, Röda Korsets Sjukhus, Brinellvägen 2, S-114 28 Stockholm, Sweden.

143 Letter to Fr. A Kornak, 10 March 2011, signed by Dr. Derek Gribbin and Dr. Dirk Kruse for Hoechst GmbH, copy in possession of the authors.

the drug itself. We freely admit that we cannot prove this conclusively, but the circumstantial evidence on this point certainly provides food for thought.

There are, though, also other plausible explanations for how thalidomide came to Chemie Grünenthal and also for how the patent specification was so detailed in relation to effects on humans. Perhaps the most compelling revolves around one of the central characters in this story, whom we have encountered several times already, Professor Werner Schulemann. After all, he was a prolific inventor of pharmaceutical compounds; Mückter had been trained by him; and Keller, the co-patentee of the original thalidomide patent, arrived at Chemie Grünenthal only shortly before that patent was filed directly from the University of Bonn (where he had worked under Schulemann's tutelage). This is all suggestive, if a bit vague. There is once again much more evidence to support this contention, though, although again we have to provide some background, and this time it stretches quite far back. For, in fact, already during the 1920s, while he was still employed as a scientist at Bayer/IG Farben, Schulemann pioneered in research and development of two extremely important families of drugs: piperidines and those based on phthalic acid. Both had close associations with thalidomide as well as other key connections. Let us look at each in turn.

Nowadays, piperidine appears on the short United Nations list of 'chemicals frequently used in the illicit manufacture of narcotic drugs and psychotropic substances',[144] but when Werner Schulemann and his team filed one of the earliest piperidine derivative patents in 1927, it seems they thought there was probably more commercial potential in dyeing cloth blue rather than getting people 'high'.[145] Soon thereafter, though, there were examples of piperidine derivatives being patented for possible unspecified pharmaceutical applications, and by 1935 scientists of Hoffman LaRoche had identified some 2-4 Dioxopiperidines which were effective sleeping drugs, or 'strong hypnotics' as they are described in the patents.[146] By the early 1940s the focus for the

[144] United Nations, 'United Nations Convention against Illicit Traffic in Narcotic Drugs and Psychotropic Substances' (1988) p. 22, available at: *www.unodc.org/pdf/convention_1988_en.pdf* <viewed 28 November 2014>.

[145] USA 1,752,617 for: Werner Schulemann, Fritz Schonhofer, and August Winkler of Elberfeld (Bayer), referencing German patents 52,228; 52,229; and 52,230 (all 1925) and US patent 1,747,521; filed in Germany 25 January 1927; Pharmaceutical products; blue dye shades.

[146] Germany 634284, 18 June 1935, German patent 634285 29, August 1935, German patent 637385, 5 September 1935, all for Hoffman LaRoche.

use of these products had moved to a very specific range of effects on the human body.

Schulemann remained closely linked to these developments. For instance, in January 1941, a team led by Dr. Rudolf Tschesche working for Schering AG in Berlin – this was a time when Schulemann was closely linked to this firm – formulated a piperidine derivative which they described as a 'spasmolytic',[147] meaning that it acts to relieve or reduce muscle spasms. What is more, Dr. Otto Eisleb of the Hoechst division of IG Farben was the lead inventor of a prominent piperidine-derived painkiller, Pethidine, in 1939. While working for IG Farben at Hofheim, furthermore, Eisleb filed a series of piperidine-derivative patents in the late 1930s, and in May 1942, he filed one that stated that the compound was a good spasmolytic as well as a painkiller (analgesic).[148] Similar piperidine derivative patent applications were made by other IG Farben scientists. Dr. Gustav Ehrhart, for instance, also of the Hoechst division, filed another in December 1942, as well as a spasmolytic and painkiller piperidine drug in the same month.[149]

Shortly after the end of World War II, a flood of piperidine-derivative patents was filed on behalf of companies closely connected with IG Farben, particularly Bayer, and also CIBA. Appendix 2 lists an illustrative sample of patents for piperidine derivatives registered between 1927 and 1953, the year prior to initial patenting of thalidomide, covering more than 290 different compounds either for IG Farben group companies or companies with very close connections to IG Farben, and particularly its Bayer division, but also Schering AG, a non-IG Farben German chemical company. Here, it is worth noting that the original English-language patent specification for thalidomide characterised it as '3-phthalimido-2,6-dioxopiperidine',[150] i.e. a piperidine derivative. In other words, far from thalidomide being a 'new type of product', it was in fact derived from a long and well recorded process of the development of chemical compounds, which lends credence to

[147] Germany 872 045 for Schering AG Dr. Rudolf Tschesche, Berlin-Wilmersdorf, Dr. Hermann Fox, Berlin-Frohnau und Dr. Karl Junkmann, Berlin. Verfahren zur Herstellung von Abkommlingen des 4-Oxypiperidins filed 15 January1941, Spasmolytic.

[148] Germany 752 755 for: I G Farbenindustrie, 19 May 1942 Dr. Otto Eisleb, Hofheim (Taunus) A G; Verfahren zur Herstellung von 1-Alkyl-4-(m-oxyphenyl)-piperidinverbindungen Good Spasmolytic and painkiller.

[149] German Patent 897561 29 December 1942, Dr. Gustav Ehrhart Hoechst, Verfahren zur Herstellung von 4-Aryl-N-alkyl-piperidin-4-carbonsäurenitrilen und – estern, spasmolytic and analgesic.

[150] UK 768821; USA 2830991.

the idea that it may well have been developed outside of Chemie Grünenthal and before 1954, with Werner Schulemann, one of the most active researchers in this family of drugs, a prime suspect for its discovery and transmission to the firm.

But Schulemann was also involved in research on another closely related family of pharmaceuticals, again since the 1920s. Indeed, a patent filed in 1926 by Werner Schulemann and his team entitled 'Manufacture of New Pharmaceutical Products'[151] discussed the use of phthalic acid. The relevance of this patent is that several of the alternative chemical names of thalidomide include 'phthalimide'.[152] This patent evidences a link among piperidine research, phthalimide and potentially also thalidomide in the person of Werner Schulemann. When considered together with his wartime work with phthalimides and his pre-war and wartime research and development of piperidines, plus the fact that he taught both Heinrich Mückter and Herbert Keller, there is a strong likelihood that Schulemann played a central role in the Grünenthal thalidomide story.

There is one more scenario to consider carefully. It has been hinted at already, and it is also probably the most controversial of those we are putting forward for how it was that thalidomide was patented with extensive indications of its impact on human beings without any evidence of prior testing. This scenario involves the potential connection between the development of nerve gases and related antidotes during the Nazi period on the one hand and thalidomide on the other. Here again, background is essential.

In early 2008, retired solicitor Jonathan Stone, a passionate campaigner for justice for the thalidomide survivors, unearthed the fact that Dr. Otto Ambros, former chief of the nerve gas development programme in Nazi Germany, had been a director of Grünenthal. What is more, even though it was quickly determined that Ambros took up this post only in the 1970s, well after the withdrawal of thalidomide in 1961, further investigation revealed links between him and Grünenthal

[151] USA 1,760,781 for Winthrop Chemical Company 20 December 1926, Werner Schulemann, Fritz Schonhofer, and August Wingler. Phthalimides.

[152] Alternative names for thalidomide include: 1H-Isoindole-1,3(2H)-dione; 2-(2,6-dioxo-3-piperidinyl)- N-(2,6-dioxo-3-piperidyl)-(6Cl,7Cl,8Cl); 1,3-Dioxo-2-(2,6-dioxopiperidin-3-yl)isoindoline; 3-Phthalimidoglutarimide; N-(2,6-Dioxo-3-piperidyl)phthalimide; N-Phthaloylglutamimide; NSC 527179; NSC 66847; α -(N-Phthalimido)glutarimide; α -N-Phthalylglutarimide; α -Phthalimidoglutarimide.

stretching back to the 1950s.[153] This suggested the possibility that the drug – which was explicitly characterised in the original patent outlined earlier in this chapter as being an anticonvulsant, acting to control muscle spasms, among other things – may in some way have come to Grünenthal as a result of wartime work on nerve agents carried out or overseen by Ambros and, more importantly, wartime work on nerve agent antidotes. This in turn set us on the trail of looking for patents of compounds similar to, but predating, thalidomide, and also for patents filed by chemists known to have been associated with Grünenthal, again predating thalidomide.

How, though, to find them? Here we had the good fortune that Michael Howard, one of the few surviving members of the T-Force that had entered Germany as the war was ending to investigate developments in science, technology and medicine that had taken place there during the Nazi period,[154] learned of our work and offered to help us out. He recommended that we investigate the reports of the Combined [British and American] Intelligence Objectives Subcommittee (CIOS), which, along with the documents seized by the T-Force and other technical investigation teams and their notes on activities undertaken while they were in Germany, are now stored in the former NAAFI club at the Imperial War Museum's Battle of Britain airfield at Duxford, in Cambridgeshire. That is where we went to uncover whatever we could find about the scientists who we knew had been connected with Grünenthal, and the range of compounds that were similar in nature and effects to thalidomide.

153 Ambros and Hermann Wirtz sat on the Supervisory Board of Knoll AG in 1960. See Knoll A.G., *Geschäftsbericht 1960.* Ambros also admitted to having been a consultant to The Distillers Company, which must relate to the late 1950s and early 1960s since this was the only time that TDC was involved in the chemical/pharmaceutical industry. See Otto Ambros to J. Peter Grace, Jr. (W.R. Grace & Co.), 30 January 1980, and James W. Nance (White House) to Congressman Tom Lantos, 13 April 1982, citation from Ronald Reagan Library, from set of documents cited by Annie Jacobsen; *Operation Paperclip;* p. 419. Copy of document in possession of authors. Christian Wagemann, who began working at Grünenthal in 1973, reported that, although Ambros officially became a member of the company's supervisory board in 1976, Ambros had been active with the company since he had started working there and, based on conversations Wagemann had with work colleagues, since even before that. Interview with Christian Wagemann by Monika Eisenberg and Martin Johnson, 7 July 2009, Aachen.

154 See Sean Longden, *T Force: the race for Nazi War Secrets, 1945* (London: Constable, 2009). Michael Howard was an advisor to Longden for this book. See also John Gimbel, *Science, technology and reparations: exploitation and plunder in postwar Germany* (Stanford: Stanford University Press, 1990); and Matthias Judt and Burghard Ciesla, eds., *Technology transfer out of Germany after 1945* (Amsterdam: Harwood Academic, 1996).

Some of the reports provided us with more detailed information about the activities of some of the notorious cast of characters who populate the pages of this book. One report, for example, detailed some of the wartime research activities of Heinrich Mückter at the Army Institute for Typhus and Virus Research in Kraków in the General Government.[155] We also found a report confirming that Werner Schulemann had, in the course of Nazi-era experiments, synthesised various phthalimide compounds, at least one of which (an attempt to combine a barbiturate molecule with a phthalimide) had a nearly identical composition and structure to thalidomide itself.[156]

Some of the reports, though, brought new characters into the frame, although this occurred in part because of connections between these characters and those we knew well already. For example, there is a full account in Duxford of an interrogation of IG Farben's Dr. Gerhard Schrader, who told investigators about how he came to invent first Tabun and then Sarin, the devastating nerve agents, under the direction of none other than Otto Ambros, who is mentioned specifically. In subsequent research, Schrader went on to invent another 65 variants of Sarin.[157] Meanwhile, in several other centres in Germany, teams of scientists were put to work on nerve agent research, development and production.[158] What is more, human testing of nerve gases on prisoners and concentration camp inmates took place at a number of locations, including IG Farben's Elberfeld laboratory and its Dyhernfurth manufacturing facility, which was under the charge of Ambros. Indeed, Ambros (who was given control not just over his company's, but also, from 1942, of Germany's overall chemical weapons development effort), along with Hitler's personal physician Karl Brandt, observed a group of concentration camp prisoners being exposed to a nerve agent in the experimental gas chamber at Bayer's Elberfeld laboratory. They

155 CIOS Target Number 24/241, 'Institut für Fleckfieber- und Virusforschung des Oberkommandos des Heeres,' by Joseph Smadel, Hans Schlumberger, and Eugene Soles, Medical Section, HQ ETOUS, 27-30 April and 16-17 May 1945. Dr. Heinrich Naeckten [sic] is listed as co-assistant leader of the Institut (p. 5), but this is clearly a transcription error, as is clear from the list of reports that were co-authored by Heinrich Mückter listed on p. 16.

156 CIOS Item No. 24 File No. XXIII-17 1946 Professor Doctor Werner Schulemann Malariologist, esp. p. 14.

157 BIOS Final report No. 714 Item No. 8 'The Development of New Insecticides and Chemical Warfare Agents' by Gerhard Schrader.

158 Nerve agent research centres included the Bayer laboratories at Leverkusen and Elberfeld, the Army Ordnance Office in Berlin, the Gas protection laboratory at Spandau, the proving ground at Raubkammer, the institute of chemistry of the Kaiser Wilhelm Institute (KWI) for medical research, Heidelberg, and major production factories at Dyhernfurth and Falkenburg. Jonathan B. Tucker, *War of Nerves: Chemical Warfare from WW1 to Al-Qaeda,* pp. 25-69.

died as a result. At the Dyhernfurth factory overseen by Ambros, where Tabun and Sarin were manufactured in large quantities, more than 3,000 Auschwitz prisoners were used as slave labour, and many died as a result of exposure to the nerve agents.[159]

These were horrible weapons of mass destruction that caused agonising death to those exposed to them for purposes of experiment and product development or in the course of manufacturing them. But it is a real mercy that they were never used by the Germans in combat during the Second World War. Precisely why this was the case is not entirely clear, although we can certainly dismiss the possibility that it was for moral or humanitarian reasons. Instead, it probably had to do with two things: fear that the Allies might have developed similar or even worse nerve agents that they would use to retaliate in the case of a German nerve gas attack; and/or the shortage (or complete lack, at times) of suitable antidotes. After all, the military problem posed by the potential use of nerve agents in combat was this: while the new nerve gases were some of the most potent weapons of mass destruction yet invented, without effective antidotes they would be as likely to kill your own troops as those of the enemy.

This is where we come back to the possible thalidomide connection with nerve-gas antidote research. In order to develop effective antidotes to these chemicals, the mechanism of action of nerve gases had to be understood, and intensive work on this began in 1943, when Professor Richard Kuhn, a chemist based at the University of Heidelberg who had been awarded the Nobel Prize for chemistry in 1938, was tasked with investigating this problem. In conjunction with this, Kuhn's team experimented with a range of products that might serve as new nerve agents, which included quinine and the Rhône-Poulenc drug Antergan.[160] Similar research took place at the University of Marburg under the direction of the Military Medical Academy, Berlin.[161]

Certainly, from 1941 Kuhn was exploring several compounds in the course of his nerve agent research to find out those which could oppose the actions of B-complex vitamins, and one at least was an analogue of

159 Jonathan B. Tucker, *War of Nerves: Chemical Warfare from WW1 to Al-Qaeda,* pp. 61-62, 44, 94,70.

160 Florian Schmaltz, *Kampstoff-Forschung im Nationalsozialismus: Zur Kooperation von Kaiser-Wilhelm-Instituten, Militär und Industrie* (Göttingen: Wallstein Verlag, 2005), p. 503.

161 The drugs that have been identified as tested by Kuhn's team are: Arecoline, Ephedrine, Atropine, Scopolamine, Lobeine, Adrenaline, Morphine, Quinine Pilocarpine, Bridal and Antergan. Florian Schmaltz, *Kampstoff-Forschung im Nationalsozialismus: Zur Kooperation von Kaiser-Wilhelm-Instituten, Militär und Industrie,* p. 463.

a thalidomide metabolite which could antagonise folic acid[162] (which was similar to Aminopterin). This work is thus a strong candidate for supplying the information which appeared in 1954 on the thalidomide patents.[163]

By early 1944, Kuhn and his team discovered the way nerve agents operated, using the neurotransmitter acetylcholine and the enzyme cholinesterase. The Team subsequently discovered SOMAN the most potent of all German nerve agents. For its part, acetylcholine is essential for the function of the parasympathetic part of the autonomic nervous system as well as the peripheral nervous system, while cholinesterase, on the other hand, breaks down acetylcholine, thus stopping its action. Nerve gases cause their toxic effects by causing the build-up of excessive acetylcholine in the body, with death accompanied by agonising muscle spasms.[164] It was determined that Atropine was effective against Sarin and Tabun poisoning precisely because it blocked the action of acetylcholine.

Even before this action was fully understood, however, efforts to develop drugs that would serve as effective antidotes were stepped up. Here, the work hinged on a continuation of an already well-developed research programme on piperidine derivatives that started in the late 1920s with work by – once again – Werner Schulemann. Appendix 2 provides a review of patents for piperidine derivatives filed by IG Farben companies or those closely connected with them (including Hoffman LaRoche and CIBA) between 1927 and 1953. While investigation of their pharmaceutical properties was clearly a goal here from the outset, it is telling that, beginning in 1941, not long after the development of the nerve agents Tabun and Sarin, the patents show that more specific neurological properties of these compounds were being identified. Already in that year, anticonvulsant effects were first reported for piperidine derivatives, which had the potential to alleviate

[162] vitamin B9.

[163] Specific compounds explored by Kuhn included N-(4-aminobezoic) glutamic acid, an analogue of the thalidomide metabolite N-(2-carboxybenzoic) glutamic acid. Duxford, FDX 890, IG W-Elberfeld Dr. Ernst Auhagen, laboratory report months April-May 1941, 'Versuche über Wirkstoffe bei Mikroorganismen', p. 4126-4133 (1-8), in particular p. 4130; also BIOS XXV-54, pp. 93-95, (Auhagen) and FIAT review of German Science No. 16 Biochemistry Part IV (main author Richard Kuhn) article: Ernst Friedrich Moller and Friedrich Weygand p. 146; Schmaltz, Florian, *Kampstoff-Forschung im Nationalsozialismus: Zur Kooperation von Kaiser-Wilhelm-Instituten,* Militär und Industrie, p. 484 f.; J.W. Faigle, H. Keberle, W. Riess, and K. Schmid (CIBA Basel) (1962) 'The Metabolic Fate of Thalidomide', *Experientia,* Vol. XVIII – Fasc 9 pp. 389-397 15 September 1962.

[164] Jonathan B. Tucker, *War of Nerves: Chemical Warfare from WW1 to Al-Qaeda,* pp. 51-54.

the most dramatic symptom of nerve gas poisoning, muscle spasms. Research and development on piperidines continued apace throughout the rest of the war and into the early post-war period, although when the actions of acetylcholine and cholinesterase were discovered by Kuhn in early 1944, this family of chemicals became redundant for nerve gas antidote research per se. By then, the actual mechanism of action of the antidote Atropine was finally understood, and it had nothing to do with anticonvulsant action or other effects described for the piperidines. Still, though, research on the piperidine family of chemicals continued, and the effects described in many of the patents for piperidine-derived pharmaceuticals filed in the late 1940s and early 1950s even began to introduce comparisons with Atropine followed by recording of a 'parasympatholytic' effect, in other words using language along the lines of that used in the original English-language thalidomide patent. Werner Schulemann's interest in this field of chemistry spanned the entire period, with his first patent for piperidines filed in 1927, and the latest, for a piperidine derivative insecticide, filed in 1955.[165]

Conclusions

So where does all of this leave us?

First of all, we freely admit that we cannot prove that thalidomide was *not* invented at Chemie Grünenthal by Herbert Keller and Willi Kunz in 1954. But we have demonstrated in this chapter that it is doubtful that it was, for several reasons: the timing of the company's decision to enter the sedative market as well as of Keller's arrival at the company in relation to the filing of the first thalidomide patent; the low level of qualifications of Kunz; and the detail given in the patent on the effects of the drug on human beings when there had been no time for any research to determine this and when claims about the testing done after the patent was filed were not only extraordinarily rudimentary, but also exclusively on animals (and on rodents for the most part).

This strongly suggests, then, that thalidomide was discovered outside of Chemie Grünenthal and prior to 1954. Here, we have offered a number of possible scenarios to explain where and when that discovery may have happened, each based on circumstantial evidence, to be sure, but each also nevertheless plausible given the network of

165 German Patent 953,878 for: BASF, Ludwigshafen dated 12 May 1955, inventors Dr. Friedrich von Bruchhausen, Dr. Werner Schulemann, Dr. Heinrich Pasedach, Dr. Otto Hertel: Insecticide.

people and organisations involved and their well-documented patterns of interest and behaviour. It is possible that the drug originated at Rhône-Poulenc, which had close ties during the war with Heinrich Mückter, Grünenthal's chief scientist by 1946, ties that continued – and indeed seem to have become even closer – after Mückter joined the staff of Chemie Grünenthal after the war. Moreover, and more importantly, the French firm licensed the brand name Contergan to Grünenthal, which was then used in Germany to market the drug. Secondly, we have suggested that the drug originated from research done by or under the direction of Professor Werner Schulemann from the University of Bonn. Finally, we have suggested it may have originated in conjunction with research on possible new nerve agents that were developed just prior to and during the war in Germany.

It is worth pointing out, too, that these three explanations are not mutually exclusive. Indeed, although it is speculative, all three of these scenarios might together provide the full explanation: Werner Schulemann may have come upon thalidomide while doing research in connection with his ongoing work on piperidines and pthalic acid derivatives; the intellectual property was then lodged with Rhône-Poulenc towards the end of the war to prevent it falling into the hands of the T-forces; and it was eventually passed on to Chemie Grünenthal. Regardless of whether or not this constitutes the full explanation, it is extremely likely that thalidomide originated in Schulemann's laboratory based on a number of facts: his longstanding interest in thalidomide-like compounds; his connections to Schering, IG Farben and Otto Ambros; his mentoring and tutoring of both Mückter and Keller; and the very narrow time frame involved between Keller's arrival at Chemie Grünenthal from the University of Bonn and the filing of the original thalidomide patent.

However, it is clear that each of these potential explanations has something to recommend it, and each has its drawbacks. But, unlike the creation myth for thalidomide propagated by Chemie Grünenthal and widely accepted in the literature since then, some of these scenarios help explain 'how they knew' about some of the effects of the drug on human subjects, while other scenarios suggest explanations for how it was that 'they did not know enough' about specific processes or varieties of drug K17.

All speculation aside, there is no doubt about this: thalidomide was unleashed on the world in the late 1950s, with dire consequences from the outset, turning rapidly into a catastrophe of momentous proportions.

Figure 8: Kevin Donnellon, aged 4.
Kevin has always maintained his enthusiasm for driving, even though the conversions needed to drive his van cost more than many supercars.

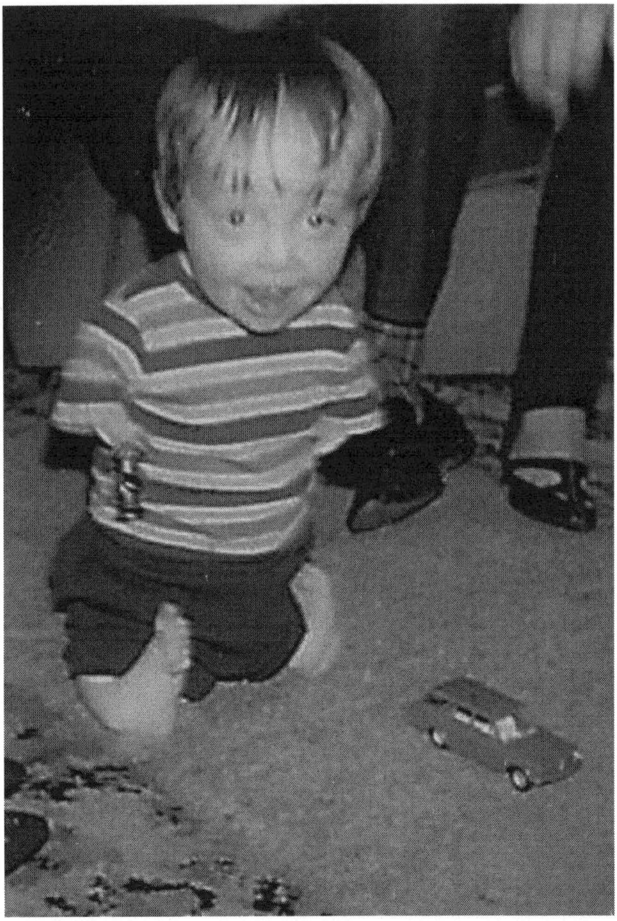

© Thalidomide Society on behalf of the copyright holder

CHAPTER FIVE

Grünenthal is 'Very Sorry'![166]

Thalidomide cover-up and conspiracy from market entry to 'withdrawal', 1957-1961.

Introduction

EVEN BEFORE THE FORMAL INTRODUCTION of thalidomide onto markets in Germany and elsewhere in 1957/58, the first babies with birth defects had been born to mothers who had taken the drug, including one case of the wife of a Chemie Grünenthal employee in Aachen. That number escalated rapidly in the next few years in line with the drug's increasing popularity, a popularity that translated into massive profits for the firm and its licensees as well as its chief scientist, Heinrich Mückter. During the entire period in which the firm sold the drug, Mückter's basic salary remained unchanged at DM 14,400 a year, a modest but respectable income. But the bonus payments he received, linked to the sales of products under his control, made him very wealthy indeed. From 1951, for instance, even well before the introduction of thalidomide, he was receiving bonuses of DM 100,000 annually on the basis of the company's sales. But this annual bonus increased by 70% when Contergan sales began in earnest in 1958. Two years later, in 1960, his bonus reached DM 270,000 and in 1961 it was DM 325,000. The firm and its owners, the Wirtz family, profited even more handsomely. By 1960, thalidomide sales accounted for half the company's turnover – about DM 20 million annually.[167]

[166] *http://www.bbc.co.uk/news/health-19443910* <viewed 14 March 2013>.

[167] Der leitende Oberstaatsanwalt bei dem Landgericht Aachen, 'Anklage gegen Wirtz u.a., Contergan-Verfahren', 10 March 1967, pp. 3-4.

That income, of course, dropped precipitously with the withdrawal of the drug from general sale in late 1961. At the same time, the firm and its senior employees faced recriminations in public and the threat of criminal charges, which eventually was realised in the form of an indictment and criminal trial, which we will look at in detail in Chapter 6. Just now, however, we need to look closely at just how much the company knew about thalidomide's devastating effect, and when, between the introduction of the drug to the market and its eventual withdrawal, kits managers came to know about it. To do this, we use archival documents prepared by prosecution staff, some of which were not introduced into court, as well as documents and testimony from the trial itself. We also use documents released by the firm under 'discovery' in conjunction with a recent class-action suit in Australia.

What we scrutinise most critically here is the repeated insistence by Chemie Grünenthal and its representatives from the time the thalidomide disaster became widely known in late 1961 that they had – and could have had – no idea that the drug might be harmful, and that the terrible 'side effects' of it were therefore completely unexpected. They have continued to assert this to the present day, as for example in conjunction with the company's public statement of regret for the disaster that was issued on 31 August 2012. Widely reported around the world at the time, the BBC website gave this account of the event and of the reaction to it among thalidomide survivors in the English-speaking world:

> *The German company that invented thalidomide has issued its first apology in 50 years to thousands of people born with disabilities after their mothers took the drug ... Grünenthal said it was 'very sorry' it had remained silent on the issue.*
>
> *But ... [the] apology [issued by the company's CEO, Harold Stock] has been dismissed as insufficient by victims' groups who say the firm should pay compensation.*[168]

The reasons that survivors remained unhappy after the speech become clear if we look at parts of the rest of it, in particular the following statement by Stock. As quoted in a report in the *Telegraph,* Stock said:

> *The thalidomide tragedy took place 50 years ago in a world completely different from today. The international scientific*

[168] *http://www.bbc.co.uk/news/health-19443910* <viewed 14 March 2013>.

community, the pharmaceutical industry and governments, legislators and administrations have had to learn a lot from it. Throughout the world the tragedy influenced the development of new authorisation procedures and legal frameworks, which seek to minimise the risks of new medicines for patients as much as possible.

Grünenthal has acted in accordance with the state of scientific knowledge and all industry standards for testing new drugs that were relevant and acknowledged in the 1950s and 1960s. We regret that the teratogenic potential of thalidomide could not be detected by the tests that we and others carried out before it was marketed.[169]

While it is true that the thalidomide disaster did prompt improvements in drug safety procedures around the world, the second paragraph of this extract from Stock's statement, which reiterates the firm's position from November 1961 onwards, is simply not true.

What we will show in this chapter is, first, that in fact Chemie Grünenthal definitely knew about the association of the drug with polyneuritis (damage to the peripheral nervous system[170]) even as early as 1956, before it was brought to market, with repeated and increasingly frequent reports coming to its attention in the late 1950s and early 1960s. The company either issued misleading or untrue responses to these reports, or simply ignored them. Second, we will show that the company knew about birth defects arising from use of the drug later, but still well before its eventual withdrawal in November 1961. Again, the response until then involved evasion, deceit and denial. Finally, we will demonstrate conclusively that the company and its senior staff *should have suspected potential impacts on unborn babies from the start,* not least because scientists and regulators in many counties raised concerns and acted with corresponding caution. In other words, the scientific knowledge and standards prevailing in many places at the time the drug was introduced were entirely adequate for

169 *http://www.telegraph.co.uk/health/healthnews/9513858/Grunenthals-thalidomide-apology-in-full.html* <viewed 14 March 2013>.

170 A number of terms have been used in our various sources for the injury to the peripheral nervous system caused by thalidomide; these include Polyneuritis, Polyneuritides, Paraesthesia, Peripheral Neuropathy (sometimes abbreviated to neuropathy), which all relate to the same set of symptoms.

preventing the disaster, but they were unfortunately either not put into practice or were simply ignored, with catastrophic results.

The introduction and withdrawal of thalidomide

After test marketing in the Hamburg area in 1956, thalidomide was launched in Germany under the Contergan brand name on 1 October 1957 and in several other countries under a variety of brand names not long after. Advertised as a 'completely safe' sedative, the drug was targeted at providing a safe alternative to barbiturate sedatives, the dangers of which included addiction and often fatal overdose. Sales grew rapidly and soon accounted for almost half the company's turnover. However, in autumn 1961, Professor Widukind Lenz in Germany and Dr. William McBride in Australia independently attributed to thalidomide the epidemic of deformities in newborns that appeared in the wake of the drug's introduction in their respective countries, leading to its withdrawal at the end of November and beginning of December 1961 in most of the countries where it had been commercially available.[171]

However, while the work of Lenz and McBride was undoubtedly crucial by virtue of serving as the proximate cause for the drug's withdrawal, the fact was that the alarm they raised formed only the last in a long series of warnings stretching back to before the drug went on the market, which Grünenthal and its licensees managed to ignore, suppress or evade. These warnings focused on two separate areas: polyneuritis, or nerve damage; and damage to unborn babies that resulted in death or, if the child survived, malformation. Although the two areas were ultimately related and although there is some overlap in chronological development in relation to each of them, it will be useful in terms of clarity to examine each in turn, not least because some of the issues they raise differ from one another.

POLYNEURITIS: EVIDENCE OF DAMAGE AND DANGER FROM THE START

There is clear and incontrovertible evidence that Dr. Heinrich Mückter was aware of the possibility of nerve damage from taking thalidomide from spring 1956 at the latest – in other words more than a year before the drug went on the market – and probably earlier. During

[171] Henning Sjöström, Robert Nilsson, *Thalidomide and the power of the drug companies,* pp. 37-68.

March and April 1956, Mückter exchanged letters with a Dr. Piacenza, who had been conducting clinical trials of thalidomide on his patients. Piacenza complained that K17 (thalidomide) had not lived up to its non-toxic billing, and indeed caused a range of side effects. He noted that there was 'absolute intolerability' among some patients taking the drug and that it had furthermore caused paraesthesia (a type of peripheral nerve damage) in one patient. Dr. Piacenza noted that despite Dr. Mückter's claim that K17 could treat tuberculosis, it was in fact completely unsuitable for TB patients because of its toxicity. He concluded by saying that a striking feature was that after taking the drug for 14 days, all patients experienced considerable pruritus, a rash that spread over the whole of the body. As a result of all of these problems, Dr. Piacenza's clinic had stopped all therapeutic treatment with K17. Writing back on 3 April 1956, Dr. Mückter told Piacenza that his reports of all of these side effects and problems were different from anything received in tests over the course of about two years in many clinics and various sanatoria. Astonishingly, though, in an apparent contradiction to what he had just written, Dr. Mückter then volunteered the information that in his view, long-term use of heavy doses of K17 produced a 'disturbance in the nervous system'. And in fact, these effects are entirely consistent with the descriptions of the effects of the drug described in the many patents for thalidomide filed by Chemie Grünenthal starting in 1954.[172]

In any event, reports flowed in regularly to the company from physicians noticing unexpected reactions to treatment with thalidomide, with their frequency and numbers increasing markedly with the ever more widespread use of the drug. By 1959, this had become a torrent. Typical of these was an inquiry on 7 October 1959 from Düsseldorf neurologist Dr. Ralph Voss, who wrote to Grünenthal to ask if the firm was aware of any information to suggest that Contergan might lead to damage to the peripheral nervous system. The company sent one of its sales representatives, Johannes Zila, to see him. In a follow up letter dated 17 December 1959, the company told Voss that:

> *...at the moment we do not have any idea how these polyneurites can be triggered by Contergan ... Considering the large number of patients who meanwhile have been regularly*

[172] Dr. Piacenza to Dr. Mückter, 25 March 1956, summary and extracts from document in Affidavit of Michael Magazanik as to the Plaintiff's case against the first defendant, Supreme Court of Victoria at Melbourne, SCI 2011 3527, 13 July 2012, pp. 18-19.

taking the preparation for 1-2 years and do not present with any disorders, however, one would have to determine that this may be an extreme occurrence – assuming it is really the effect of Contergan.[173]

This might appear to be a reasonable reply, but only if it were indeed true that there had not been any previous reports of this type of problem with Contergan. It most certainly was not, as we have seen already. Moreover, in the months immediately prior to and also just after Dr. Voss' report, we have other examples not only of reported problems, but also of false denials that the firm had received any previous such reports:

- On 14 July 1959, sales representative Zila, the same person who would later visit Dr. Voss, submitted a report to the company indicating that a Dusseldorf pharmacist had notified him of several cases of constipation and one of paraesthesia (nerve injury, peripheral neuritis) that had potentially developed from Contergan, noting the pharmacist's observation that perhaps the drug had an effect on circulation.
- Then on 27 August 1959 a Swiss company, Pharmacolor AG, reported that 20 'renowned doctors' had reported severe side effects with Softenon (another trade name for thalidomide) after as little as one tablet of Softenon Forte, including severe tiredness, trembling hands etc.
- On 15 October 1959, just a week after the first letter from Dr. Voss, the sales team reported two more cases of sensory disturbances in toes and fingers following Contergan use.
- A week after that, on 26 October 1959, the company wrote to a doctor in Iserlohn who had reported a case of sensory disturbance following Contergan use saying there had been no reports of any similar cases.
- Not long after, Dr. Graf von Schroder reported two female patients with paraesthesia in their calves. On 30 December

[173] Quotation from letter from Grünenthal to Dr. Voss, 17 December 1959, which is a follow-up to 'Grünenthal report by sales rep Zila', 17 December 1959, extracts in: Affidavit of Michael Magazanik as to the Plaintiff's case against the first defendant, Supreme Court of Victoria at Melbourne, SCI 2011 3527, 13 July 2012, p. 25.

1959, the company wrote back to him denying they had ever heard of paraesthesia following Contergan use.[174]

One final example of this remarkable pattern of behaviour from early 1960 is particularly harrowing. In a letter of 11 March 1960, responding to complaints from a surgeon, Chemie Grünenthal wrote:

> *Thank you for your letter of 8th March 1960 in which you tell us you are increasingly suffering from paraesthesia and hypoaesthesias on your hands and feet which are being seen as probable polyneuritis by a specialist of internal medicine.*
>
> *You are enquiring if such symptoms could possibly be due to the regular use over approximately seven months of two tablets of Contergan Forte prior to going to sleep since no other cause for the emergence [of these symptoms] has so far been found.*
>
> *We wish to advise you that we have received no such reports to date. This is despite the fact that the use of Contergan has been growing steadily over several years so that we can draw on extensive experience with this product by now.*[175]

A surgeon who can no longer feel his fingers and feet has come to the end of his surgical career. The likelihood is that the person affected never recovered, even if he had ignored this false reassurance and stopped taking the tablets straight away.

These examples represent just a small sample of such reports, which, taken together, demonstrate clearly a consistent pattern of duplicitous and mendacious corporate behaviour during a period of just eight months of the five years in which thalidomide was sold widely.[176]

But the reports did not stop there. Instead, they continued and, what is more, some of those involved became more active and systematic in their reporting. After being brushed off by the company, for example, Dr. Voss proved more persistent than most. Far from accepting the company's response, he followed up with more reports of cases of nerve

[174] Extracts of these documents are summarised and/or translated and reproduced in Affidavit of Michael Magazanik as to the Plaintiff's case against the first defendant, Supreme Court of Victoria at Melbourne, SCI 2011 3527, 13 July 2012, pp. 24-26.

[175] Letter from Grünenthal to surgeon, 11 March 1960, extract of translation of document in: Affidavit of Michael Magazanik as to the Plaintiff's case against the first defendant, Supreme Court of Victoria at Melbourne, SCI 2011 3527, 13 July 2012, pp. 26-27.

[176] Various documents from the period summarised and/or translated/reproduced in: Affidavit of Michael Magazanik as to the Plaintiff's case against the first defendant, Supreme Court of Victoria at Melbourne, SCI 2011 3527, 13 July 2012, pp. 24-27.

damage in the next few months, and others joined him in alerting the company to the dangers of polyneuritis posed through long-term use of the drug.[177] In December 1960, Voss began a systematic survey of similar cases. Unknown to him and other doctors and specialists outside the company, by the end of 1960, at least 1,600 such reports had been submitted to the company.[178] Dr. Voss presented his findings, using several case reports of polyneuritis, to a postgraduate course for neurologists in Dusseldorf on 15 February 1961. The company got advance warning of this event and sent a high-ranking employee, Dr. Sievers, to visit Voss beforehand to try to persuade him to play down the effects of Contergan in his lecture. Voss refused, not least because there was ample evidence by then that thalidomide caused toxic polyneuritis: when taken continuously for periods of between two weeks and three years, the effects would start to appear, first as a prickly feeling in the extremities followed by numbness which usually began in the toes. The numbness then spread to the ball of the foot, to the ankles and subsequently to the calves, but did not usually extend above the knee. Sometime later, though, it would start to affect the tips of the fingers and then the hands. After this, severe muscular pains and cramps began in the extremities, involving weakness of the limbs and disturbances of the reflexes and coordination of the arms and legs, which often made walking difficult, not least because balance was affected. In a significant number of particularly unfortunate cases, this eventually led to partial paralysis and permanent disability.[179]

By early 1961, ever-increasing reports of thalidomide's role in causing nervous system injuries led to probing questions from Grünenthal's licensee companies and critical reports in the medical and scientific press. Still, though, Chemie Grünenthal's rearguard action continued. For one thing, the lies kept coming: the firm continued to deny that thalidomide was causing nervous system damage, and it continued to maintain that it had never had more than the tiniest number of reports of such damage. Company officials also continued to try to fob people off systematically. In February 1961, in a response to an inquiry from Richardson Merrell, Grünenthal's prospective (and ultimately unsuccessful) US licensee company, about information the

[177] Medizinisch Pharmazeutische Studiengesellschaft e.V., Dokumentation III/71, 'Schriftlicher Einstellungsbeschluß der Ersten Großen Strafkammer des Landgerichts Aachen im sog.' Contergan-Verfahren' (Frankfurt, 1971), pp. 44-45, quotation from p. 44.
[178] Henning Sjöström, Robert Nilsson, *Thalidomide and the power of the drug companies,* p. 64.
[179] *Ibid.,* pp. 52-53.

Americans received from the Food and Drug Administration (FDA) arising from the recent publication of an article in the *British Medical Journal* describing thalidomide-induced nerve damage, the German firm claimed that it only ever received one report of nerve damage after thalidomide use. It further contended that it had had no word from Distillers about the information that had led to the findings published in the article.[180]

Grünenthal's managers focused, in addition, on trying to win scientific support in Germany, and placed their hopes on articles about thalidomide due to be published in German medical journals in April or May of 1961 which they thought would be positive. Just to be sure, though, they explored the possibility of 'doctoring' the results of studies, to produce a bias in favour of thalidomide – methods planned included weeding out reports where the Contergan connection was not 'certain' (which allows a lot of scope for eliminating unfavourable reports), and also devising a questionnaire survey with questions formulated to favour Contergan. They furthermore considered commissioning a market research centre to do a poll on soporifics, in the hope that this might show Contergan in a favourable light. At one company meeting on 22 March 1961, they even went as far as discussing the possibility of commissioning research into whether thalidomide acted as an anti-vitamin, blocking the activity of those B-vitamins known to be involved in the operation of the nervous system, but the probable cost of DM 250,000 was felt to be prohibitive unless this could be justified in relation to sales figures.[181]

If all else failed, though, they were prepared to use blunter instruments. Dr. Mückter hired Ernst Gunther Jahnke, a private detective, to try to discredit some of the doctors making adverse reports about Contergan. On one occasion, they even 'smuggled' a woman into the clinic of one doctor, to see what happened if she pretended to have Contergan polyneuritis.[182] This was a sign of desperation as well as

[180] Chemie Grünenthal (Leufgens and von Schrader) to Richardson Merrell (Dr. Murray), 27 February 1961, in Affidavit of Michael Magazanik as to the Plaintiff's case against the first defendant, Supreme Court of Victoria at Melbourne, SCI 2011 3527 dated 13 July 2012 pp. 42-44.

[181] Extracts of documents summarised and/or translated/reproduced in: Affidavit of Michael Magazanik as to the Plaintiff's case against the first defendant, Supreme Court of Victoria at Melbourne, SCI 2011 3527, 13 July 2012, pp. 32-36, 44-48.

[182] Henning Sjöström, Robert Nilsson, *Thalidomide and the power of the drug companies,* pp. 69, 92; *The Sunday Times* Insight Team, *Suffer The Children: The Story of Thalidomide,* pp. 39-40.

ruthlessness though, and it appears as if senior staff members at Grünenthal were, by spring 1961, gradually realising that the jig was up. On 29 March 1961, they consulted their insurance company (Gerling) in relation to the potential product liability complaints. By July, the Grünenthal legal department was addressing the possibility that the insurers might refuse cover, but even if they did not refuse, they ascertained that the maximum cover under the policy was only DM 500,000. The firm's legal team then started exploring patient records and trying to construct arguments that would exonerate the company's behaviour through late 1960. The team hoped that the liability could be limited to a total of 46 claims starting in autumn of 1960, but company officials feared there in fact might be around 4,000 claims, which could cost between DM 12 million and DM 18 million to settle.[183]

From all of this, it is clear that Chemie Grünenthal knew by spring of 1956 at the latest, well over a year before thalidomide was introduced to the market, that it had toxic side effects, especially in higher doses. The response to a raft of reports of nerve damage following the use of the drug, though, was to deny or to downplay the reports, something that demonstrates particularly high levels of callousness and irresponsibility given that the company also continued to claim that the drug was safe for pregnant women and children. This was true even for several months after senior managers consulted their insurers about product liability claims, an action that implied that they knew that the reports they were receiving were credible and that legal action was about to be taken.

Damage to children: The pattern was clear long before autumn 1961

The first baby with thalidomide damage was born in Aachen on Christmas Day 1956 to the wife of a Chemie Grünenthal employee. That fact was, of course, determined much later in the aftermath of the withdrawal of the drug from general sale on 27 November 1961. This withdrawal in turn was in direct response to an article in the *Welt am Sonntag* newspaper on Sunday, 26 November 1961 reporting the research findings of Professor Widukind Lenz from earlier that month, which concluded that thalidomide was responsible for the epidemic of

[183] Summaries and translations of extracts of documents in: Affidavit of Michael Magazanik as to the Plaintiff's case against the first defendant, Supreme Court of Victoria at Melbourne, SCI 2011 3527, 13 July 2012, pp. 93-109.

malformations in newborns in Germany (and of course in other countries where the drug was sold).[184] And, as we have noted earlier in this chapter, from the date of the withdrawal of the drug to the present, Chemie Grünenthal has consistently maintained that this was 'an unforeseeable tragedy' and that the company withdrew the drug as soon as it became aware of its connection to birth defects.[185] We will reject the first part of that claim decisively and systematically in the next subsection, which focuses on what others knew and acted upon before the withdrawal of the drug. To begin with, though, we take issue with the second part of the claim: Grünenthal's senior managers were in fact aware of the likelihood of the link between pregnant mothers taking the drug and malformations in their babies well before 1961.

Indeed, there were reports suggesting this connection as early as 1958. US-based pharmaceuticals firm Smith Kline & French had begun testing thalidomide some time before that with a view to selling it under licence from Grünenthal. The company's investigations eventually concluded by 1958 that the drug was ineffective as a sedative, and the company decided for that reason not to proceed. But there was an additional reason for the American firm's reluctance to go forward with purchasing a licence for the drug: August 1958 test reports produced by the firm mentioned one, possibly two, babies with birth defects born following tests on 875 people including pregnant women.[186] This information, which Chemie Grünenthal would certainly have been aware of, was disregarded.

Let us concede that there is perhaps a (vanishingly small) possibility that the German company was not aware of Smith Kline & French's findings from summer 1958. There is, however, no question that by 1959, company personnel were alerted about suspicions about the link between the drug and birth defects. One report came from Dr. Randolph Riemschneider, a Berlin-based German scientist who was at the time doing specialised research on amphibians in Brazil. After

[184] *The Sunday Times* Insight Team, *Suffer The Children: The Story of Thalidomide,* pp. 97-105.

[185] Chemie Grünenthal, *1946-2006: 60 Years of Grünenthal* (Stolberg, 2006), p. 9.

[186] Claim filed 9 August 2012 in Philadelphia County Court of Common Pleas states documentary evidence of testing by Smith, Kline and French in 1956 showed thalidomide useless as a sedative, and one, possibly two babies with birth defects born to women in August 1958 among a group of 875 people who took the drug during testing: *http://www.hbsslaw.com/resources/newsroom/hagens-berman-files-new-lawsuit-on-behalf-of-11-alleged-us-thalidomide-victims* <viewed 13 March 2013>. See also Gero Gemballa, Der dreifache Skandal; 30 Jahre nach Contergan. Eine Dokumentation, 1993, Luchterhand Literaturverlag GmbH, Hamburg, pp. 46-47.

testing the effects of thalidomide on tadpoles during 1958 and 1959, Riemschneider concluded that there was a possible link between birth defects observed and the ingestion of the drug, a link that required further research. As he later wrote:

> *May 1959 – Teratogenic effects were observed in some cases on frogs and photographed at the end of metamorphosis ... As we had no experience in the fields of embryopathy and teratogenicity, these observations were not accorded the significance they deserved. But [nevertheless] ... we sent this information with photos to Chemie Grünenthal, the manufacturers of thalidomide, in Jun 59 ... requesting funds for a doctoral candidate. Unfortunately, no answer was forthcoming at the time.*[187]

But already in spring 1959, there were credible and alarming reports to the firm from closer to home of the drug's devastating effects, not on tadpoles, but on newborn humans. On 19 March 1959, the wife of a Dr. Kreideweiß gave birth to a baby who had ear and eye defects. Because there was no history of birth defects in his and his wife's respective families, and because he could think of no other possible cause, he suspected that the damage may have resulted from his wife having taken thalidomide. Shortly thereafter, Kreideweiß discovered two other cases of babies with birth defects whose mothers had taken thalidomide. In April 1959, he reported his suspicions to Dr. Mannheim of Grünenthal, who was a personal friend of Kreideweiß. Mannheim testified later (in 1970) at the criminal trial of the company's executives that he remembered speaking to Kreideweiß in 1959 about the possible effects of the drug on babies in the context of Kreideweiß's malformed child and two other cases. Mannheim, however, contended in his testimony at the trial that if this conversation had taken place, '...he could not imagine that ... he would not have informed the Stolberg headquarters', and he was therefore convinced that the discussion had not occurred. The prosecutor noted, however, that Dr. Kreideweiß had remained adamant under oath that his version of events was accurate.[188]

187 Randolph Riemschneider (2004) 'Thalidomide A remedy with two faces', *The BWW Society; the Institute for the Advancement of Positive Global Solutions* Nov/Dec Issue 2004.

188 Testimony and prosecution questioning of Dr. Mannheim (Grünenthal wissenschaftlicher Aussendienst), 211. Verhandlungstag 9.3.1970: Dagmar and Karl-Heinz Wenzel; *Der Contergan-Prozess* vol. V; p. 69. Mannheim's version of events presented at the trial contradicts what he stated in response to questioning from prosecutors who were preparing for the trial in

There is stronger evidence still that the firm knew very well about suspicions of a link between thalidomide and birth defects by summer 1961 at the very latest – in other words, months earlier than Grünenthal staff claimed was the case. In a statement made to the prosecution in May 1963, Jacques Künzli, who had been a sales representative of Chemie Grünenthal, claimed that the firm's Dr. Werner had indicated in September 1961 that 'much more serious damage was to be expected [from thalidomide] than was known already. He meant by that damages other than polyneuritis'. Künzli went on to indicate that Dr. Werner specifically pointed at that time to a need to do research on animals to determine 'whether damage to the foetus might be possible'. He noted, in addition, that his recollection was that 'Dr. Mückter had said that this would have to be looked into'.[189]

There is, moreover, additional testimony in support of this from another employee of Grünenthal. Dr. Günther von Waldeyer-Hartz, a chemist who worked for the company briefly in 1961, wrote to the Justice Ministry of North Rhine Westphalia from his new home in Berkeley, California, on 5 January 1969, stating that:

> *In the second half of October [1961] I, together with four other members of the training course for drug representatives [Aertztebesucher], had the opportunity to have a look at the production facilities of Chemie Grünenthal.*
>
> *When we did so, a packaging machine for thalidomide was shown to us which had packages with a sticker attached stating:*
>
> *'...not for pregnant women.'*[190]

In other words, there is no question about the fact that there were early and credible reports to Chemie Grünenthal of a suspected link between thalidomide and malformations in newborns, but, just as in the case with reports about polyneuritis caused by the drug, they were ignored. Before we go on to consider the compelling evidence that

1964. Here he made it clear that he and Dr. Kreideweiß had indeed discussed cases of children born with birth defects, including Dr. Kreideweiß's own son, the cause of which may have been thalidomide. He did, though, indicate that he did not consider the conversation important enough to report to his company, Chemie Grünenthal. Vernehmung Dr. Mannheim, 17 December 1964, LAV NRW R, Gerichte Rep. 139 Nr. 175 Bl. 110/8/8.

189 Vernehmung Jacques Künzli, 6 May 1963, LA NRW Duisburg, 175 093-094.

190 Waldeyer-Hartz to Justizministerium Düsseldorf, 5 January 1969 (Abschrift), LA NRW Duisburg, Ger Rep 0139-00276-0006-0008. Quotation from 0006. Emphasis in original.

Chemie Grünenthal personnel should in any case have suspected that there might be a causal connection between ingestion of the drug and birth defects, recall what we considered at some length in Chapter 1: it is a sobering fact that, had any of these early reports been acted on, even if only in the form of providing a clear warning to expectant mothers and their doctors of the potential dangers of thalidomide, then the vast proportion – possibly as many as 95-99% – of the babies destroyed or damaged by the drug would not have been harmed.

DAMAGE TO CHILDREN: THEY SHOULD HAVE SUSPECTED IT – AND EVEN *EXPECTED* IT

Not only should Chemie Grünenthal have taken the reports suggesting a link between pregnant mothers taking thalidomide and malformations in their babies seriously from 1959 at the latest, company officials should actually have *anticipated* them long before that on the basis of scientific knowledge that was already well developed by the mid-1950s. There are at least three ways that this could and should have happened, two of which Grünenthal staff knew about from direct experience and one of which anyone working at the time who had any specialist knowledge of pharmaceuticals and their side effects should have known about. Let us look at each in turn.

The first way in which damage to children should have been anticipated was through the fact that it was very quickly recognised that the drug suppressed thyroid activity, with some of the consequences of such suppression being well known in the medical/pharmaceutical community. For instance, the results of one set of tests in autumn 1957, commissioned by the Distillers Company in the UK prior to the start of sales of the drug in that country, represented an unambiguous and direct warning in this regard. Carried out by Drs. J.McC. Murdoch and G.D. Campbell of Edinburgh University and Edinburgh Royal Infirmary respectively, with the help of Professor D.M. Dunlop and Dr. A.G. Macgregor, the results were published on 11 January 1958 in the *British Medical Journal.* This paper raised serious questions about the safety of thalidomide (K17):

> *In Germany clinical experience has already led to the suggestion that the drug is virtually non-toxic and will prove valuable in various psychological disturbances such as anxiety states, mild depression, excitability, and some vegetative dystonias (Esser*

> *and Heinzler, 1956; Jung, 1956; Stark, 1956). These workers [sic] observed marked reduction of the raised basal metabolic rate in mild and moderately severe cases of hyperthyroidism as the result of K 17 therapy. From the results obtained it appears that N-phthalyl glutamic acid imide has a mild but definite antithyroid activity when given in doses of 200 mg. or more. At present the mode of its action is unknown. In the meantime, therefore, it would seem unjustifiable to use the drug for long-term sedative or hypnotic therapy, pending the results of a more detailed study of its long-term effects in a larger series of patients, and notably those suffering from mild or moderately severe hyperthyroidism.*[191]

Distillers' staff members were aware of the test results prior to publication, not least because they had commissioned the study, and these would have been reported to Grünenthal, although Dr. von Schrader Beielstein from Grünenthal indicated in a telephone conversation with Dr. Murray of Richardson Merrell in the US that the company 'did not know about the information provided by Distillers on neuritides'. However, von Schrader Beielstein did his best to calm the potential licensee in America, again stretching the truth to its limits, and came away from the phone call with the impression that 'this conversation has lifted the negative perception of us [on the part of the Americans] which was caused by the British publication [in the *British Medical Journal]* and our "silence" so far on these cases.'[192] In this regard, it was significant that the *British Medical Journal* report did not mention Distaval (the principal UK brand name for thalidomide), instead referring to the drug generically as K17, Grünenthal's internal designation for thalidomide and its derivatives. This was quite possibly owing to pressure placed on the authors of the *British Medical Journal* piece by Distillers.

This was important. After all, physicians in Britain and elsewhere who read this article may not have known that what was referred to as K17 was the active ingredient in Distaval and therefore did not realise the potential implications of prescribing it for use by pregnant women.

191 J. McC. Murdoch, G.D. Campbell (1958) Antithyroid activity of N-Phthalyl Glutamic Acid Imide (K 17) in *BMJ* (11 January 1958); p. 84.

192 Memo by Dr. von Schrader re. telephone conversation with Dr. Murray at R-M, 28 February 1961, summarised in Affidavit of Michael Magazanik as to the plaintiff's case against the second and third defendants, Supreme Court of Victoria at Melbourne, SCI 2011 3527, 13 July 2012, p. 44.

If they had known, however, they would have been very wary of doing this. Staff at Distillers and Chemie Grünenthal, on the other hand, had no such excuse. They knew what K17 was, for one thing; and, what is more, the dangers of reduced thyroid activity were widely known long before this time, especially with respect to pregnant women and babies. Indeed, already in the middle of the 19th century, reduced thyroid activity had been linked to what was then known as 'cretinism' (a contemporary term for a serious learning disability). Furthermore, it was well-known that pregnant women with reduced thyroid activity were more likely to lose their babies – possibly arising from foetal thyroid deficiency.[193] By 1953, testing of the drug thiouracil had demonstrated beyond any doubt the risk of thyroid suppression to the foetus.[194]

What is more, the knowledge that thalidomide suppressed the thyroid gland would not have come as any surprise at all to Grünenthal staff; the action of the drug in reducing the metabolic rate of the body (a key effect of reduced thyroid gland output) was implied in the first patents of K17 from 1954, and was actually stated explicitly in their Austrian thalidomide patent of 1956.[195] Nevertheless, although Murdoch and Campbell noted that thyroid suppression was evident at doses of 100-200 mg, this was in fact the very dose suggested by Grünenthal and Distillers when Softenon Forte and Distaval Forte went on the market. (Each tablet of these contained 100 mg of thalidomide, with a recommended dose of one to two tablets.[196] Two tablets of Contergan Forte, by the way, was also the exact dose that was being taken each night by the surgeon mentioned earlier in the chapter who reported his Contergan-induced polyneuritis to the company.)

Further information about this effect emerged in 1960 in a paper summarising thyroid research since 1936, focusing in particular on a number of studies from the early 1950s that showed the range of effects

[193] C.A. Aldrich (1936) 'Growth and Development: the Endocrine Glands and Growth (Continued) The Thyroid', *The Journal of Pediatrics* Vol. 8, Issue 3 pp. 381-389 March 1936; J.R. Bloss (1937) 'The Importance of Routine Thyroid Study in Prenatal Care', *Southern Medical Journal* Vol. 30 No. 6 pp. 637-639, June 1937.

[194] N. Elphinstone (1953) 'Thiouracil in pregnancy; its effect on the foetus', *The Lancet,* pp. 1281-1284 June 27 1953; D. Morris (1953) 'Transient Hypothyroidism in a Newborn Infant', *The Lancet* p. 1284 June 27 1953.

[195] Osterreiches Patentamt *Patentschrift nr. 193880,* application date 31 January 1956 'Verfahren zur Herstellung von neuen Amino-piperidin-2,6-dionen'. Inventors: Dr. Dr. Herbert Keller, Dr. Wilhelm Kunz.

[196] Softenon and Softenon Forte instruction literature supplied in the packaging with the tablets (copies in M.J. Archive).

the thyroid gland has on the brain and central nervous system. It suggested that the fact that reduced thyroid output had more severe effects in the foetus and small children than in adults 'may be due both to a direct, though as yet undefined, relationship between thyroid hormone and neural maturation, and to the secondary influence of thyroid deficiencies on other tissues'.[197] In other words, the developing nervous system in the foetus was thought to be particularly vulnerable to damage, which could possibly be caused by a change in the levels of thyroxin produced by the thyroid gland.

Overall, then, medical knowledge established in the 19th century was supplemented by a mass of evidence produced during the 20 years prior to the release of thalidomide, with the later research in particular indicating that anything that suppressed the production of thyroxin, the hormone made by the thyroid gland, might interfere with the developing brain and nervous system and thus kill or damage the unborn child. Grünenthal and its UK licensee, Distillers, which commissioned the work, completely ignored the recommendations and possible implications of Murdoch and Campbell's study. This was no small or inadvertent oversight.

The second way in which it should have been suspected that there might be a connection between thalidomide and birth defects involved the drug's anti-vitamin activity, a report on which arrived at Grünenthal in November 1959 at the latest.[198] There is no doubt that Grünenthal officials must have known about the report's implications immediately on the basis of direct experience with another drug that it had sold under licence since the early 1950s, Aminopterin.

Before we look at that other drug, though, let us consider the November 1959 report, which was from Dr. Michaels, a Grünenthal employee, who wrote in his monthly submission to company headquarters that a Dr. Wowalka had been studying the mechanism of action of K17 and considered that this mechanism was an anti-glutamic acid one.[199] According to an expert report prepared for the prosecution in July 1965, by Professor Josef Kimmig, this finding should immediately have rung alarm bells for anyone with a medical

[197] J.T. Eayrs (1960) 'Influence of the Thyroid on the Central Nervous System', *British Medical Bulletin* 1960 pp. 122-126.
[198] Monthly report by Dr. Michael November 1959 (Gerichte Rep 139 No 21 157), LA NRW Duisburg.
[199] *Ibid.*

background and experience. As Professor Kimmig, who was also an expert witness in the later trial, explained in his expert report:

> *Glutamic acid is one of three components of folic acid, and the various known folic acid antagonists always act against just one of these three components.*

He went on to name a thalidomide metabolite, 'alpha amino glutamic acid imide', as a probable glutamic acid antagonist, and therefore a folic acid antagonist. He stressed, furthermore, that this action had been known to be teratogenic since 1949-1950.[200]

This was not an obscure finding and, what is more, there is no question about the fact that *key staff at Chemie Grünenthal knew this very well from their own experience.* After all, one of Grünenthal's products which the company had sold under licence in Germany since 1953 was Aminopterin, which had been developed and was 'owned' by Lederle laboratories in the USA.[201] A key property of this drug was that it blocked the action of folic acid in the body, which was thought to be useful in treating cancer, as a possible way of stopping the growth of tumours. It was, however, well known that if given to pregnant women Aminopterin would often cause miscarriages and birth defects.[202]

The scientific research and evidence behind this knowledge was extensive well before thalidomide was introduced commercially. Moreover, one early study was particularly suggestive, although admittedly based on a small number of participants in a somewhat bizarre experiment: in the early 1950s, J.B. Thiersch administered Aminopterin to 12 pregnant women who were considered to be in need of therapeutic abortions. As a result, ten of the babies died through miscarriage or stillbirth, and the two others who were born alive

200 Prof. Dr. Med. J. Kimmig to the Lead Prosecutor of the Landgericht Aachen, Betr.: Ermittlungsverfahren gegen Hermann Wirtz u.a., 12 July 1965, LAV NRW R, Gerichte Rep 139, Nr.6 Bl.06354-06358. Kimmig's testimony at the trial is summarised briefly in Dagmar and Karl-Heinz Wenzel; *Der Contergan-Prozess* vol. III, p. 165. The summary of the testimony does not include any of the detail given in the affidavit.

201 Aminopterin was the property of Lederle Pharmaceuticals (USA). In the Grünenthal company history *Der Eigene Weg* produced in 2006 for the firms' 60 anniversary: 'Ab 1953 führte Grünenthal alle Lederle Produkte ibn Deutschland ein, bis Lederle sie 1959 in eigene Organisation in Deutschland überführte.'

202 T.H. Jukes, A.L. Franklin, E.L.R. Stokstad (1950) 'Pteroylglutamic acid antagonists', *Annals of the New York Academy of Sciences,* Vol. 52 pp. 1336-1341, July 1950. Also, C.C. Stock, J.J. Biesele, J.H. Burchenai, D.A. Karnofsky, A.E. Moore, and K. Sugiura (1950) 'Folic Acid Antagonists and Experimental Tumours', *Annals of New York Academy of Sciences,* Vol 52 pp. 1360-1378 July 1950; J.B. Thiersch (1949) 'Bone-Marrow Changes in Man after treatment with Aminopterin, Amethopterin, and Aminoanfol', *Cancer,* September 1949, pp. 877-883.

suffered major malformations; three of the dead babies had multiple malformations as well. Futhermore, these effects occurred at very small dosage levels of 6-12 mg administered over the course of just 2-5 days.[203] A subsequent study, reported in a 1955 paper, undertook a much larger-scale investigation of this effect on rat embryos. High dosage rates produced a high level of foetal death, sometimes up to 100%. Lower levels produced an extensive range of birth defects, which included fused or multiple digits, skeletal anomalies including damage to fore and hind limbs and damage to internal organs including the uro-genital organs, cardiovascular system and kidneys, as well as damage to facial structures – in fact, a range of defects and malformations similar to those produced in humans by thalidomide.[204]

Again, there is no question that Grünenthal knew about this and its implications; after all, the drug used to produce folic acid deficiency in the animals experimented upon in the research behind this 1955 report was Aminopterin. Indeed, as Thiersch claimed in response to questions posed by the prosecutors preparing the trial of Grünenthal executives in February 1968, this action and its potential effects were more generally known by 1959 on the basis of a range of well publicised scientific experiments that took place between 1949 and the late 1950s. He went on:

> *Thalidomide is similar in its chemical structure to folic acid antagonists ... The molecule was therefore to be suspected of having an effect on the foetus.*[205]

The third means through which Grünenthal should have suspected that there might be a connection between thalidomide and foetal malformations involved the drug's potential for neurotoxic (nerve poisoning) effects. This, too, was on the basis of scientific knowledge already well established at the time. The scientist charged with examining the application of Richardson Merrell company to the American FDA for approval to distribute thalidomide in the United

[203] J.B. Thiersch (1952) 'Therapeutic abortions with a folic acid antagonist, 4-aminopteroyl-glutamic acid (4-amino P.G.A) administered by the oral route', *Am. J. Obst. & Gynec.* 63(6): pp. 1298-1304.

[204] M.M. Nelson, H.V. Wright, C.W. Asling, H.M. Evans (1955) 'Multiple Congenital Abnormalities Resulting from Transitory Deficiency of Pteroylglutamic Acid During Gestation in the Rat', *Journal of Nutrition* 56(3): 349-69 (11 July 1955).

[205] Answers of John B. Thiersch MD to questions from prosectors from NRW, 20 February 1968 (translation), LA NRW Ger Rep 0139 00367a, Bl. 0002-0010, quotation from p. 9 of document (Bl. 0010).

States, Dr. Frances Kelsey, for instance, had her suspicions about the drug's neurotoxic potential aroused by an article in the *British Medical Journal* on 28 January 1961 entitled 'Is Thalidomide to Blame'.[206] The article reported five cases of neuropathy following treatment with thalidomide and triggered a long-running series of similar reports from doctors in Britain. Her concern was that if the drug was a neurotoxin, which was looking more and more likely given this report, it would also very probably harm the foetus. Kelsey had learnt about this general problem in the early 1940s while working as a pharmacologist involved in malaria research. Quinine was the original drug used to treat malaria, and it is highly neurotoxic. Given to a pregnant rabbit, quinine harms the embryos by killing them or malforming their eyes and ears. Kelsey knew that if a drug with similar effects to quinine were taken by a pregnant woman, there was a risk her unborn child could be similarly killed or damaged. Kelsey had also been part of a team in 1938 that investigated the toxic properties of a drug that had caused at least 107 deaths, a tragedy that triggered passage of much more stringent drug approval laws in the United States than was the case elsewhere at that time.[207]

Again, this was specialist knowledge, of course, but not rocket science even at the time for those working as academics or industry practitioners in the area of pharmaceuticals. As Kelsey wrote in 1965:

> *...when the thalidomide application was under study there was developing an increasing interest in the effects of the drugs and other environmental hazards on the human fetus and newborn, all of which contributed to our caution in evaluating the application.*

Furthermore, she noted specifically research showing risks of birth defects published in 1940 on the effects of the German measles virus

[206] E.V. Kuenssberg, J.A. Simpson, J.B. Stanton, 'Is Thalidomide to Blame', *BMJ* 1961; 1:236 (Published 28 January 1961).

[207] Bren, Linda (2001) 'Frances Oldham Kelsey: FDA Medical Reviewer Leaves Her Mark on History', *FDA Consumer* 35(2):24–29 'Frances Oldham Kelsey, who saved U.S. babies from thalidomide, dies at 101', *New York Times* (7 August 2015), available at: *http://www.nytimes.com/2015/08/08/science/frances-oldham-kelsey-fda-doctor-who-exposed-danger-of-thalidomide-dies-at-101.html?_r=0* <viewed 26 October 2015>. Evidence on quinine is also available from *http://www.fda.gov; http://www.resource4defectivedrugs.com/topics/quinine.html* <viewed 12 May 2010>, which lists birth defects and miscarriage as possible side effects of quinine.

and a paper published in 1952 on the effects of – what else? – Aminopterin.[208]

The potential dangers of thalidomide: The reason the drug was not approved for sale or prescription in many countries

The story about Frances Kelsey leads us nicely into the final key point of this chapter. Whether the potential dangers of thalidomide lay in nerve damage, in foetal malformations and stillbirths or both, there is no question that the company (and the countries where the drug was approved for sale) acted recklessly and irresponsibly. We have already established that they should have known better given the state of medical knowledge at the time. This is reinforced by the fact that scientists and regulators in a number of countries acted on the basis of this knowledge to block or severely restrict sale of the drug. Their caution meant that the countries involved were largely spared the epidemic of birth defects that followed in the wake of the drug's introduction. What is more, these countries varied widely by language, culture, politics and history, and included the USA, Turkey, East Germany, France and Portugal. In other words, we are dealing with medical knowledge that was sufficiently diffused to lead many to reject applications to approve thalidomide for sale or distribution. The reasoning behind denying the applications differed somewhat for each country, although there were also a number of similarities.

In the United States, Dr. Frances Kelsey, a Canadian physician and pharmacologist, was given the task of vetting the application for approval of thalidomide for sale there as her first brief at the US FDA. As mentioned already, her suspicions were raised by the article in the *British Medical Journal* in January 1961 about thalidomide's possible neurotoxic properties as evidenced in its connection with nerve damage, combined with her experience with quinine. She also shared in the widespread concern at the time about the impact of drugs in general on babies. But it is important to underscore again, in addition, that the US differed from many other countries at the time by virtue of having a rigorous approval process in place when thalidomide was being introduced. Indeed, the very fact that there was an FDA which employed Kelsey and gave her such wide-ranging powers was unusual

[208] Kelsey, F.O. (1965) 'Problems raised for the FDA by the occurrence of Thalidomide Embryopathy in Germany, 1960-1961', *Am. J. Public Health Nations Health,* 1965 May; 55:703-7.

and can be traced back to a pharmaceutical disaster in the United States in the 1930s involving Elixir sulfanilamide, which caused at least 107 deaths. Again, Kelsey herself was part of the team tasked in 1938 with determining why the drug was harmful.

Even under the strict American drug safety laws through which Kelsey dealt with the application for approval of thalidomide at the FDA, however, she had to resist intense pressure from the prospective American licensee, Richardson Merrell. The company complained bitterly to her superiors about her repeated insistence that the company provide more information and evidence. In the end, though, she was able to delay the approval process through November 1961, when confirmation of the drug's role in birth defects effectively suspended the approval process in the United States.[209]

In Turkey, too, there was a key individual who blocked approval of the licensing of the drug there, the virologist Dr. S.T. Aygun, although the basis for his caution about the drug differed from that of Kelsey. Aygun, a vegetarian and opponent of experimenting on live animals, distrusted the testing (such as it was) reported by Grünenthal. Using a range of non-animal testing methods involving tissue cultures instead, he concluded the drug was not safe in 1960, and no licence was granted in Turkey.[210]

Another country that took a strong line against thalidomide was the German Democratic Republic (East Germany). A Grünenthal thalidomide patent application was filed there on 4 February 1956.[211] The next step involved an approval process for allowing distribution of the drug in East Germany, which did not take place for some time, although the reasons for the delay are not clear. At the beginning of 1961, scientific experts considered its possible introduction, but their considered view, based on the information provided in the patent, was that the drug

[209] 'Frances Oldham Kelsey, who saved U.S. babies from thalidomide, dies at 101', *New York Times* (7 August 2015), available at: *http://www.nytimes.com/2015/08/08/science/frances-oldham-kelsey-fda-doctor-who-exposed-danger-of-thalidomide-dies-at-101.html?_r=0* <viewed 26 October 2015>.

[210] 'The Doctor Who Prevented Thalidomide in Turkey', *Turkey Medical Tribune* (22 August 2008), p.24; Michael M.J. Fischer, *Anthropological futures* (Durham, NC: Duke University Press, 2009) p. 97; Joanne Zurio, Deborah Rudacille and Alan M. Goldberg, *Animals and Alternatives in Testing: History, science and ethics* (Johns Hopkins University Center for Alternatives to Animal Testing, 2010) chapter three, available at: *http://caat.jhsph.edu/publications/animal_alternatives/chapter3.html* <viewed 26 October 2015>. Zurio et.al. note that Aygun's claims based on tissue culture testing were never verified.

[211] DDR Patentschrift nr. DD 14567, Verfahren zur Herstellung von Amino-piperidin-2.6-dionen, inventors Dr. Herbert Keller, Dr. Willi Kunz for Chemie Grünenthal GmbH, application date 4 February 1956.

posed major risks. They noted the structure of the molecule meant that this compound might have 'unexpected effects when taken long-term', and that an 'embryo-toxic effect ... is not an unforeseeable fact, but has to be considered a possibility'. What is more, like Kelsey, the East German scientists were concerned about reports of neurotoxicity. Commenting that thalidomide had never been credited with life-saving significance, they concluded that the risks identified were not worth taking in light of limited potential benefits. But they went still further. Their concerns about the drug were such that not only did they refuse a licence, but also insisted that action be taken to prevent the drug being introduced by any private route,[212] which was extremely important in the German-German context of the first seven months of 1961 before the construction of the Berlin Wall. In any event, this constituted the most robust rejection of thalidomide recorded in any country where approval was applied for.

A patent for thalidomide was filed in France on 17 May 1955,[213] yet between then and the end of November 1961, when it was confirmed that the drug almost surely caused birth defects, no permission to distribute it was granted by the authorities. The primary reason for this lack of approval in France differed from that of East Germany or Turkey, but was similar to that of the United States: it hinged on a relatively strict regulatory regime for pharmaceuticals. Again, this was the result of a drug disaster, although it was much more recent in the case of France than it was for the US. During the period 1954-1955, a formulation error in a drug for treatment of staphylococcal infections sold under the brand name Stalinon led to the deaths of 102 'from neurotoxicity and 100 patients [were] affected by paraplegia'. French health authorities therefore intervened strongly with strict regulations announced in February 1959 that required evaluation of a drug's therapeutic effectiveness, 'its safety under normal conditions of use' and its manufacturing processes. The information that could be provided for

212 Undated statement (ca. early 1961) by the Institute for Pharmacology and Toxicology (Berlin, East Germany), translated and excerpted in Affidavit of Michael Magazanik as to the Plaintiff's case against the first defendant, Supreme Court of Victoria at Melbourne, SCI 2011 3527 dated 13 July 2012, pp. 112-114. Quotation is from p. 113.

213 France Brevet D'Invention no. 1,164,512 Procédé d'obtention de nouveaux produits de la série des amino-pipéridine-2,6-diones, for Chemie Grünenthal GmbH application date 17 May 1955.

thalidomide, of course, could not withstand such scrutiny, and the drug therefore 'was not marketed in France which was spared the tragedy'.[214]

The case of Portugal's refusal for Grünenthal's application for the rights to distribute the drug there involved, as in most of the other countries that rejected such applications, deep scepticism about the information made available about testing regimes. Evidence produced for the criminal trial of Grünenthal executives in Aachen revealed that the company's application for approval via its intended Portuguese licensee company (which planned to market it under the brand name Enterosediv) was firmly rejected in a letter dated 18 July 1960:

> *Unfortunately, the methods of study [employed] are ... utterly inadequate and for the purposes of registration completely ineligible ... You will understand that under the circumstances we will not be able to file an application for approval of the preparations (including Enterosediv) [for commercial sale].*[215]

Conclusion

Let us revisit Grünenthal's statement of 31 August 2012 in light of the evidence we have just presented. There are two serious errors of fact in it. The first is in this part of the statement:

> *...Grünenthal has acted in accordance with the state of scientific knowledge and all industry standards for testing new drugs that were relevant and acknowledged in the 1950s and 1960s.*[216]

This statement is quite simply untrue. The tests that the firm reported it had carried out in its own laboratory were rudimentary at best, and do not appear even to have involved the compound that came to be marketed as thalidomide, at least initially. The system of 'clinical trials' used by the company, moreover, seems to have involved simply passing out samples and asking for feedback (which was routinely ignored if not positive). As we have seen, other companies, organisations and individuals did much more rigorous testing. In other

214 Agnès Saint Raymond and Anthony J. Humphreys, 'Human medicinal products in the European Union: Regulations, directives and structures', p. 363, in John P. Griffin, John Posner and Geoffrey R. Barker, eds., *The Textbook of Pharmaceutical Medicine,* 7th edition (Chichester: John Wiley, 2013).

215 Der Leitende Oberstaatsanwalt be idem Landgericht Aachen, 'Anklage gegen Wirtz u.a.: Contergan-Verfahren', 10 March 1967, vol. I, p. 127.

216 *http://www.telegraph.co.uk/health/healthnews/9513858/Grunenthals-thalidomide-apology-in-full.html* <viewed 14 March 2013>.

words, the 'state of scientific knowledge and ... industry standards for testing new drugs' available at the time were *completely adequate* for identifying the potential risks associated with the drug. It is just that Chemie Grünenthal did not apply them. What is worse, when adverse feedback was received, it was generally ignored or denied, the latter often involving outright lies about an absence of previous negative reports.

However, the second part of this statement is perhaps even more shockingly misleading. The company claimed that:

> *We regret that the teratogenic potential of thalidomide could not be detected by the tests that we and others carried out before it was marketed.*[217]

As we have seen, it is indeed true that the tests carried out by Grünenthal were not capable of detecting any teratogenic risks. But the company had ample warning of this risk from testing conducted by other people and organisations, information about which Grünenthal was either provided or received directly. The tests carried out by Smith Kline & French during 1956-1958 in the USA, for instance, identified the teratogenic possibility of thalidomide. What is more, the implications of the tests carried out for Distillers by Murdoch and Campbell in late 1957 and published in early 1958 pointed strongly to a teratogenic risk associated with suppressing the action of the thyroid gland. Finally, in the following year, 1959, the company ignored reports from Dr. Kreidewiess and Professor Riemschneider that gave clear evidence of a potential teratogenic effect.

This pattern of ignoring repeated reports suggesting potential damage to babies caused by thalidomide was all the more remarkable and sickening because the company and many others must have had suspicions from the outset that there was a strong possibility of this effect. We have explored three reasons that such suspicions should have been aroused. The first of these involved the drug's effect on the thyroid gland; the second, the anti-vitamin effects of thalidomide that were similar to those of Aminopterin; and the third, the neurotoxic effects of thalidomide that were similar to compounds such as quinine.

Instead of acting on such reports and suspicions, the company responded to concerns raised by doctors about peripheral neuritis by

[217] *Ibid.*

lying not once or twice, but hundreds of times,[218] and by systematically ignoring the hazards company officials were exposing the public to. Virtually all the evidence of this behaviour presented above was available to the North Rhine Westphalia Public Prosecutor before the start of the criminal trial of Grünenthal executives in 1968. It ought therefore to have been a straightforward matter to put it before the court and secure a conviction. This would have confirmed the fears of the company's owners and given rise to claims for – and awards of – compensation at a level that would no doubt have bankrupted the company and quite possibly its sister companies owned by the same group of shareholders. Yet this did not happen, and we need to explore the reasons that it did not. The next stage in our investigation of the thalidomide catastrophe therefore involves examination of the criminal trial and the circumstances surrounding its eventual abandonment.

Figure 9: Katrina Gardner (formerly d'Andilly), aged 22 months with her mother, Pearl, on holiday in Great Yarmouth, 1964. Pearl has wrapped Katrina up out of love and protection from other people's stares.

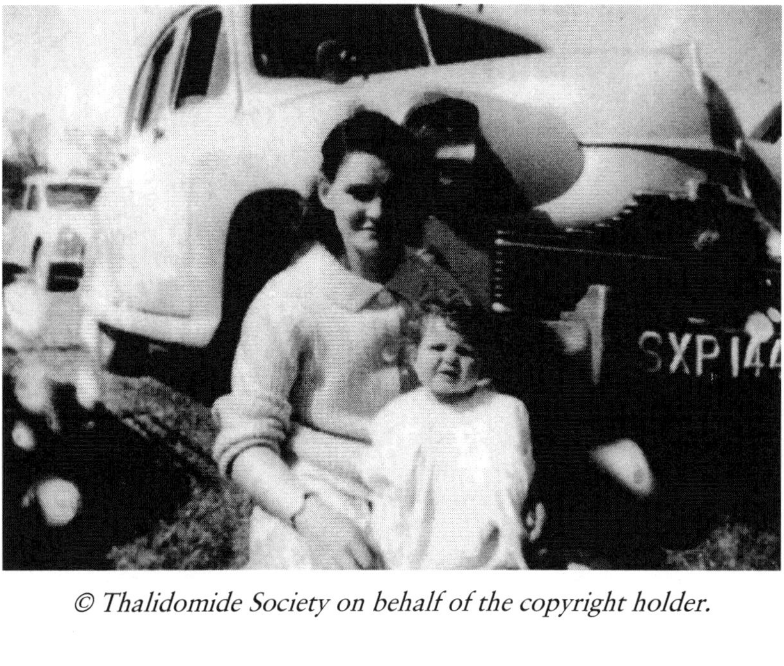

© Thalidomide Society on behalf of the copyright holder.

[218] e.g. One information mailing to doctors attempting to minimise the reported side-effects was sent to 60,154 addressees on 31 March 1961; Henning Sjöström, Robert Nilsson, *Thalidomide and the power of the drug companies*, p. 67.

CHAPTER SIX

Trying for Justice (1)

Chemie Grünenthal's executives before the court.

WHEN THE JUDGES CALLED THE CRIMINAL trial of Chemie Grünenthal executives to order on 27 May 1968, it was the second major prosecution of key employees of a German chemical firm in just over two decades. Just as in the 'IG Farben Case' that started in Nuremberg with the filing of an indictment against 23 top managers of IG Farbenindustrie AG in May 1947 (officially known as United States of America vs. Carl Krauch et al.),[219] all nine key executives of Grünenthal identified in the indictment were meant to be put on trial, although one manager in the Farben case and two (eventually three) in the Grünenthal case were excused from the main trial (and tried separately) on grounds of ill health. An additional defendant in the Grünenthal case passed away before the trial was eventually suspended. Nevertheless, there were significant similarities between the two. Both trials, for example, attracted enormous media and public attention. Both involved the collection of masses of evidence, much of which was not used in the trial itself. Both were protracted and expensive. And both featured outcomes that were and remain controversial.

There are, of course, many differences. The IG Farben trial was shorter by far: from arraignment to sentencing took just under a year.[220] In contrast, the Chemie Grünenthal trial lasted about two years and

[219] *Trials of War Criminals before the Nuernberg Military Tribunals* (TWC), vols. VII-VIII: 'The I.G. Farben Case' (Washington, DC: US Government Printing Office, 1953). Information on number of defendants, excusing of one on grounds of ill health, and dates of indictment, etc. is in volume VII, pp. 1-3.

[220] TWC, vol. VII, p. 3.

seven months. The IG Farben trial was also much bigger, in particular in terms of number of defendants and the attendant defence and prosecution staff that this entailed. Moreover, the IG Farben trial involved an American court trying German defendants in occupied Germany, whereas the Chemie Grünenthal case was a purely German affair, something that was highly significant, as we shall soon see. The two trials differed from one another, in addition, by virtue of the fact that Otto Ambros, a towering figure in the German chemical industry for much of the 20th century, was convicted in the IG Farben trial of crimes against humanity, including use of slave labour and mistreatment and murder of enslaved labourers, and sentenced to eight years in prison, whereas, as indicated in Chapters 3 and 4, he had a much more shadowy role – but a role nonetheless – in relation to the circumstances that led to the Chemie Grünenthal case. Finally, the two trials differed in this respect: not just Ambros, but a significant number of other IG Farben executives, were convicted and banned from working for the successor companies of IG Farben that were in the process of being established by the early 1950s, although one of the US prosecutors later commented that their sentences were 'light enough to please a chicken thief'.[221] In stark contrast, the case against Chemie Grünenthal executives was suspended because 'public interest in a continuation of the criminal prosecution no longer exists',[222] although in bizarre circumstances. Certainly, the outcome here could not have been more different from that of the IG Farben trial: *all* of the surviving Grünenthal trial defendants left the courtroom without a criminal record, and those who were still employees of the firm were free to go back to work there without any restrictions whatsoever.

The trial itself was covered extensively by international media, and there is even a multi-volume summary of the case as it unfolded over more than two-and-a-half years.[223] It has also been dealt with extensively in Sjöström and Nilsson's *Thalidomide and the power of the*

[221] Josiah DuBois, *The Devil's Chemists: 24 Conspirators of the International Farben Cartel who Manufacture Wars* (Boston: Beacon Press, 1952), p. 339. Cf. also Grietjet Baars, *Capitalism's Victor's Justice? The Hidden Stories behind the Prosecution of Industrialists Post-WWII*, pp. 163-193, here p. 186, in Kevin Heler and Gerry Simpson, eds., *The Hidden Histories of War Crimes Trials* (Oxford: OUP, 2013).

[222] Medizinisch Pharmazeutische Studiengesellschaft e.V., Dokumentation III/71, 'Schriftlicher Einstellungsbeschluß der Ersten Großen Strafkammer des Landgerichts Aachen im sog. Contergan-Verfahren' (Frankfurt, 1971) p. 71.

[223] There were routine reports during the trial in *Der Spiegel* and *Time*, for example, as well as in other media outlets. The summary of the trial, which includes some verbatim testimony, is in Dagmar and Karl-Heinz Wenzel, *Der Contergan-Prozess* (6 volumes).

drug companies[224] as well as in a recent PhD,[225] and we therefore do not need to go over most of this information and analysis again here. But what went on behind the scenes, what was not done and why, these are key issues that have been much less explored to date, and we will present new evidence that sheds light on many of these questions.[226] We focus here first on the decision to go to trial, the gathering of evidence and the reasons for delay in going before the court, looking in particular at irregularities that have been suggested by a number of authors, but for which we have uncovered new evidence. We then explore the trial briefly. But our main concern here involves the engineering of a suspension of the trial through political intervention and attempts to mobilise funds to that end from a number of sources, including other companies in the West German chemical and pharmaceutical industries, churches and the German federal government. Finally, we look at the content of the judges' decision on the ending of the trial and its immediate aftermath, in particular the creation of a foundation to provide aid to thalidomide-damaged children in Germany. There is mention in the judges' decision to suspend the trial of 'voluntary contributions [by the defendants] to those in need from their private funds', which was one of the reasons 'public interest ... no longer existed' in continuing prosecution.[227] And these funds, everyone knew at the time, were part of the basis for the then impending formation of the foundation, although this connection was not stated explicitly. In what follows, though, we will present evidence that the foundation and the trial's end were much more intimately connected to one another than anyone has previously suggested.

[224] Henning Sjöström, Robert Nilsson, *Thalidomide and the power of the drug companies,* Chapter 12.

[225] Niklas Lenhard-Schramm, 'Die Haltung des Landes Nordrhein-Westfalen zu Contergan und den Folgen', PhD dissertation, University of Münster, 2016, Chapter 3. This work is not just a PhD, but also constitutes a research report commissioned by North Rhine Westphalia's Ministerium für Gesundheit, Emanzipation, Pflege und Alter.

[226] Some of this evidence is examined in Lenhard-Schramm, 'Die Haltung...', and the author also details the background to the trial. The PhD appeared after a draft of this book had been completed and the evidence presented here independently compiled and analysed.

[227] Medizinisch Pharmazeutische Studiengesellschaft e.V., Dokumentation III/71, 'Schriftlicher Einstellungsbeschluß der Ersten Großen Strafkammer des Landgerichts Aachen im sog. Contergan-Verfahren' (Frankfurt, 1971), p. 71. The judges also mentioned the amount agreed to by Chemie Grünenthal, DM 110 million. See p. 74.

Figure 10: Simone Illger, about the age she was when the Contergan trial began

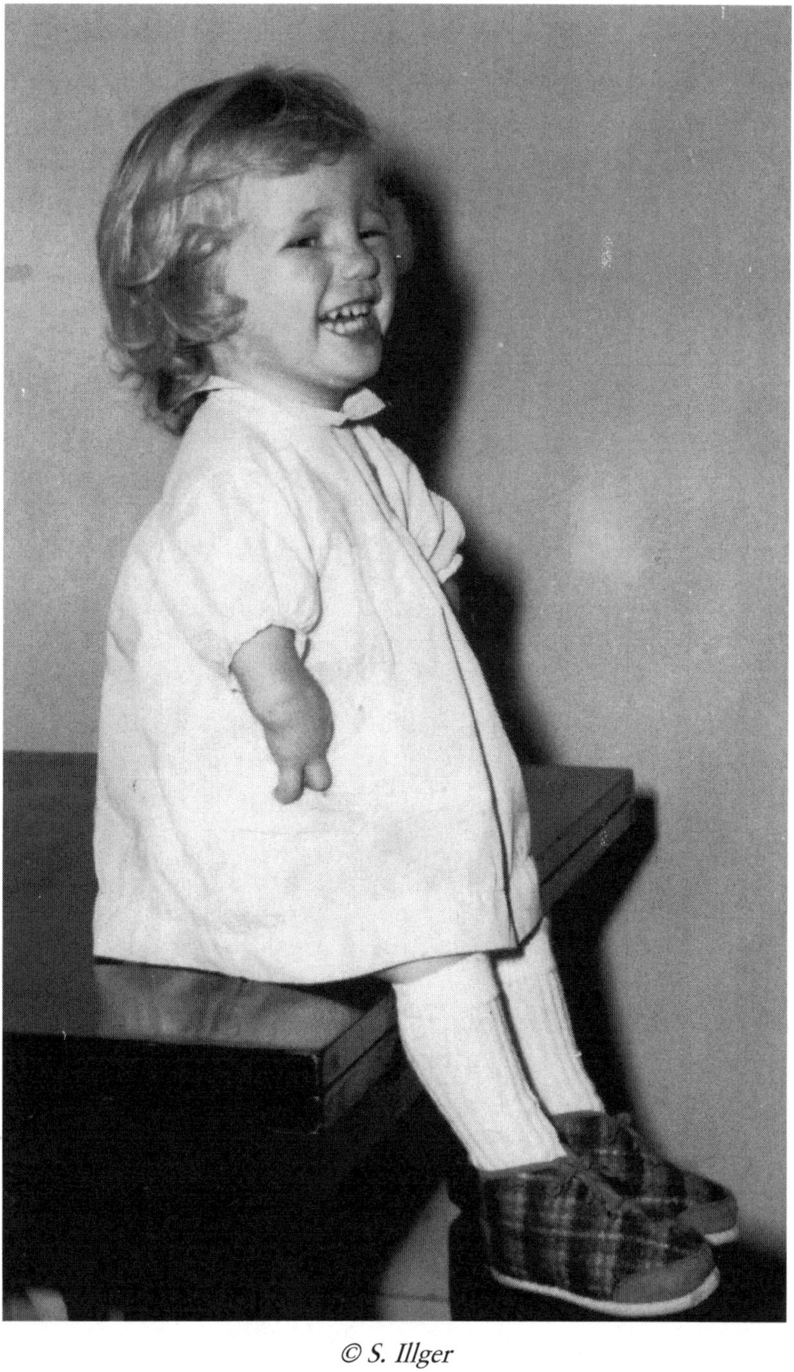

© S. Illger

Preparing for trial, and manoeuvring to avoid it

Let us start at the beginning.

Thalidomide was withdrawn from sale in Germany on 27 November 1961 in the wake of an article linking the drug to severe malformations in newborns that appeared the day before in the *Welt am Sonntag* newspaper. Not surprisingly, the search for justice, the search for someone who bore the legal and moral responsibility for the disaster and who should therefore be punished and to pay to ameliorate it in some way or another, started immediately. There were some who wanted to assign blame at a very high level indeed. For instance, later in the 1960s when the trial was beginning, *Spiegel* magazine commented:

> *Nine men have been indicted. What has not been indicted is the readiness of an era with so much trust in science as to consume medicines by the ton, despite the fact that scientists even now do not know the ways in which most medicines affect the human organism.*[228]

Spiegel's indictment of an entire generation, most would agree, was clearly overblown and far too general, and ultimately would have had the effect of letting those who in fact were responsible off the hook. In any case, it could not form the basis for legal action. In this regard, there were only two possible culprits: the German federal or state governments for not having regulated the introduction of thalidomide and other drugs effectively; and/or those who ran the company that created and produced the drug, Chemie Grünenthal. Already in 1962, the tabloid *Bild am Sonntag* accused the federal government of not doing enough for the children affected by thalidomide and called for passage of a law to compensate them. Officials at the Health Ministry and the Ministry of the Interior believed there might be grounds for a lot of pressure to be exercised on the federal government in this regard, in part because, as a Health Ministry official pointed out in an internal memo commenting on the article, at present the government 'only registers, but does not regulate' pharmaceutical trade in the Federal Republic.[229] Still, although the German federal government eventually became deeply involved in the negotiations and funding for the

[228] 'Prozesse: Contergan: Chiffre K17', *Der Spiegel,* nr. 23/1968, p. 48.

[229] Federal Ministry of Health (Schaudienst; Frandsen), 'Vermerk betr. Durchrühurung der Sozialhilfe fü Körperbehinderte, hier: Hilfe für die sog. Contergan-Kinder', 26 June 1962, BArch B106/10805.

foundation that provided aid to thalidomide victims, it shouldered precious little responsibility for some time. Again, *Spiegel* from 1968:

> *The Federal Ministry of Health has to date spent a total of 11.5 million marks in connection with the Contergan catastrophe. This contribution aided in part the expansion of specialised clinics, homes and special schools – which had been planned in any case – and in part redounded to the benefit of those engaged in the development of prosthetics and other aid implements, but it did not go directly to those who had been affected.*[230]

However, it was clear from the outset that there was a set of actors who were even more likely to be found to be liable for the havoc wreaked by thalidomide: the managers of the company that produced it. Here, action was not slow in coming. On 18 December 1961, just three weeks after the withdrawal of thalidomide from the German market, the prosecutor's office in Aachen, the city nearest Stolberg, where Chemie Grünenthal was headquartered, launched a formal inquiry into the affair with a view to possibly pressing criminal charges against representatives of the firm.

Still, although the inquiry may have started quickly, it moved forward at a snail's pace. Partly, this had to do with the sheer complexity of the case in medical and scientific terms. Prosecutors took statements and reports from hundreds of survivors and their families, as well as from medical and scientific experts and employees of the firm. They collected thousands upon thousands of pages of documents from governmental authorities and, following a raid on Grünenthal's headquarters, from the firm itself. Just to give a sense of the scale of this effort: a *selection* from the documents that the prosecution generated and collected that was put together for the actual trial amounted to 264 Leitz document boxes, 750,000 pages in all.[231]

So, yes, that all took a considerable amount of time to put together and sift through. But a crucial part of the reason that the indictment was not issued until 10 March 1967 and that the trial did not begin until more than a year after that, on 27 May 1968, was that those who were about to be accused 'lawyered up' very effectively, choosing experienced and/or well-connected attorneys to represent them.

[230] 'Prozesse: Contergan: Chiffre K17', *Der Spiegel*, nr. 23/1968, p. 48.
[231] *Ibid.*, p. 48; Der leitende Oberstaatsanwalt bei dem Landgericht Aachen, 'Anklage gegen Wirtz u.a., Contergan-Verfahren', 10 March 1967, pp. ix-xlviii.

Hermann Wirtz, for example, chose one Professor Dr. Dahs as his defence attorney to begin with, but dropped him as of 9 November 1966 in favour of the well-connected and highly experienced Dr. Dr. [sic] Josef Neuberger.[232] Frank Dahrendorf, an up-and-coming Hamburg-based lawyer with extremely good connections – his brother was Ralf Dahrendorf, a highly regarded professor, public intellectual and Liberal Democratic politician in Germany who later became head of the London School of Economics and eventually a member of the House of Lords – represented Klaus Winandi, one of the other defendants.[233] Dahrendorf later worked on behalf of some of the other defendants as well. In any event, Neuberger, Dahrendorf and the other attorneys representing those who were eventually indicted used every tactic at their disposal to kick the trial into the long grass.

But it is one thing to lawyer up – which is, after all, completely legal, even if at the same time it favours the well connected, powerful and wealthy. It is, however, quite another thing to engage in shady, semi-legal and perhaps illegal practices. Here, the extent of conflict of interest – writ very large indeed – that can be proven based on newly available documents is extraordinary.

One of the most striking examples of this involved Josef Neuberger, appointed Hermann Wirtz's defence attorney in November 1966. When he visited prosecuting attorneys Dr. Knipfer and Dr. Havertz shortly after that to inform them that he had been appointed chief counsel for Wirtz, Neuberger asked Knipfer for a written indication of the main points of the case against his client. Knipfer complied in a letter of 22 November that asked for a response by 7 December. Neuberger was nothing if not punctual. On 6 December, a 42-page commentary dated 5 December arrived at the prosecutor's office, with a cover letter from Neuberger indicating that:

> *I am of the opinion that all of the points you touched on have been exhaustively and convincingly answered therein [i.e. in the commentary] so that nothing more should stand in the way of a termination of the proceedings [against Wirtz].*

232 Dr. Havertz, 'Vermerk für die Handakten', 17 November 1966, Ger Rep 0139 00321a, Bl. 156-157, LA NRW Duisburg.

233 Der leitende Oberstaatsanwalt bei dem Landgericht Aachen, 'Anklage gegen Wirtz u.a., Contergan-Verfahren', 10 March 1967, pp. i-ii.

Later the same day, Neuberger phoned the prosecutor's office to request to meet in person. He visited the office on 7 December to speak with Knipfer and Havertz. Part of what he had to say was to be expected. Neuberger reiterated verbally that if his commentary were read 'closely and objectively', he did not see any grounds whatsoever for the prosecution of his client. But then he dropped the bombshell: he was giving up his work as defence attorney with immediate effect to assume the office of Minister of Justice for the state of North Rhine Westphalia the following day. His associate Dr. Pick would take over his duties as defence attorney for Hermann Wirtz.[234]

This is so extraordinary it deserves to be highlighted: the person who ultimately controlled the prosecution of Chemie Grünenthal executives (Stolberg, the location of the firm's headquarters, was in North Rhine Westphalia) was none other than the former defence attorney for the main accused, and he remained in the picture to a greater or lesser degree throughout the trial.[235] Indeed, from 8 December 1966 until September 1972 – which encompasses the entire length of the trial of Chemie Grünenthal executives and beyond – North Rhine Westphalian Justice Minister Josef Neuberger effectively continued to represent Hermann Wirtz through his associates in his legal partnership, Neuberger, Pick und Greeven, his name remaining on the law firm's letterhead even well after he had assumed the office of Minister of Justice.[236]

The precise ways in which he exercised this effective continuation of being a representative of the defence while at the same time Justice Minister are not entirely clear from the documents, but there are some irrefutable indications at times. On 9 February 1967, for instance, his designated secretary of state (who was to take office on 1 March), Ernst-Friedemann Freiherr von Münchhausen, called the Aachen

[234] Memorandum by Dr. Knipfer, December 1966, LAV NRW R, Gerichte Rep; 139 Nr. 321a Bl. 158-160.

[235] Lenhard-Schramm contends that Neuberger's direct influence over the trial after he became Justice Minister was minimal by virtue of the fact that the presentation of the indictment a few months later (in March 1967) placed responsibility for the trial in the hands of the prosecutors, not the North Rhine Westphalian government. (pp. 10, 506ff) Based on the evidence we present here, it is clear that Neuberger's influence on the trial after he became Justice Minister may have been indirect, but it was present and effective.

[236] Examples include Georg Greeven to I. Große Strafkammer Aachen, 'In der Strafsache gegen Wirtz u.a.', 24 May 1968, and Neuberger, Pick and Greeven, Attorneys, to Chairman of the Erste Strafkammer beim Landgericht Aachen, 'In der Strafsache gegen den Fabrikanten Hermann Wirtz', 2 May 1969, LAV NRW R, Gerichte Rep. 139 Nr. 266a Bl. 15 and Gerichte Rep. 139 Nr. 266b Bl. 216 respectively.

prosecutor's office 'on behalf of the minister' to inquire about the way the prospective trial of Chemie Grünenthal executives might be going and in particular about whether there were still plans to indict Wirtz.[237] Von Münchhausen's role as intermediary in the negotiations to suspend the trial was central, as we shall see later in this chapter. On 24 May 1968, moreover, Neuberger's practice – again, his name was still on the stationery – took over the representation of the other key defendant in the trial, Heinrich Mückter. The evidence that Neuberger continued to be involved in the case is still stronger, however: on 20 August 1968, for instance, he wrote to Dr. Erich Schmidt-Leichner, who by then served as Mückter's lead attorney, offering him legal advice.[238] More telling still, Neuberger's law partner, Pick, was designated by Chemie Grünenthal in February 1970 as a formal consultant (with the title Attorney-in-fact for the Negotiations with the Ministries) in the federal government's working group that was tasked with drafting legislation to create a foundation to administer the compensation funds that the firm would pay in order to bring the trial to an end. Pick was explicitly listed as an 'associate of Dr. Dr. Neuberger'.[239]

These certainly highly inappropriate and possibly illegal interventions by Neuberger continued during the remainder of the preparation for, and the conduct of, the trial, and the Justice Minister often worked via his close colleague (and therefore proxy), Freiherr (Baron) von Münchhausen. In the short term, pressure from another quarter required Neuberger in his new position to pay some direct attention to the Contergan case. The day he took office, the German press agency *dpa* reported that representatives of the children damaged by the drug had brought a complaint to the Justice Minister of the state of North Rhine Westphalia because they were under the impression that the Contergan case was being dragged out ('verschleppt').[240] The response is not in the file, but one can only imagine that in spite of its

[237] Memo, Havertz, 9 February 1967, Ger Rep 00139 Nr. 321 174, LA NRW Duisburg.

[238] Neuberger to Schmidt-Leichner, 20 August 1968, AdsD Bonn, Nachlass Josef Neuberger, private Korrespondenz, pages not numbered. It is not clear from the content of this letter that this advice pertained directly to the Chemie Grünenthal trial, but the technical legal issues discussed were certainly of relevance to it. Moreover, given that Schmidt-Leichner was at the time it was written taking part on a practically daily basis in the trial, and that it must have been the main focus of his work at the time, it is very likely that it pertained to the trial.

[239] Wichmann to Ministerialdirector Dahlmann et. al., 13 February 1970, and attachment; 'Gesprächspartner der Arbeitsgruppe', n.d. [February 1970], both in B141/59477. The latter document indicates Pick's title and notes that he is an associate of Dr. Dr. Neuberger.

[240] Memorandum by Dr. Knipfer, December 1966, p. 161, LAV NRW R, Gerichte Rep. 139 Nr. 321a.

clear justification, the accusation made by the children's representative was denied.

Given the fact that the deck was stacked against a trial taking place at all, it is perhaps surprising that a mere three months after Neuberger's appointment as Justice Minister of North Rhine Westphalia – remember that this is very speedy in terms of the glacial progress of the inquiry and prosecution to date – the indictment was finally put forward formally. On 10 March 1967, nine defendants were named, and they were charged with a range of felonies involving negligence leading to bodily harm through causing polyneuritis and also birth defects and malformations. In addition, they were charged with having made misleading claims in selling thalidomide. The indictment ran to no fewer than 972 pages in two volumes, with a total of 613 pages covering the indictment itself followed by 359 pages of references; these were no slim volumes. The preliminary pages (paginated in Roman numerals in volume one) pushed them to over 1,000 pages in all, naming 352 prospective witnesses for the prosecution along with 29 expert witnesses, mostly academics or medical practitioners.[241]

The indictment first gave a brief biography of each of the accused and his position within Chemie Grünenthal, followed by an overview of the key issues in relation to the state's case for a causal relationship between thalidomide and nerve damage, severe malformations in babies and other damage to humans caused by the drug. The bulk of the document, though, consisted of a detailed chronology of the alleged criminal actions as they developed during the period stretching from the patenting of thalidomide in 1954 through its introduction to the market in 1956/1957, culminating ultimately in its withdrawal in late 1961. Here, some of the evidence gathered during the long preparation for the indictment and the prospective trial was touched on briefly as the prosecution told a tale of inadequate testing; misleading advertising and claims; refusal to take on board early reports of problems with the drug; the massive income that the company derived from it; and its resistance not just to withdrawing the drug, but even to requiring it to be prescribed rather than sold over the counter. Those at the firm were

[241] Der leitende Oberstaatsanwalt bei dem Landgericht Aachen, 'Anklage gegen Wirtz u.a., Contergan-Verfahren', 10 March 1967, 2 vols. The preliminary pages involve pp. ix-xlvii of volume 1.

moreover accused of refusing to provide inserts in the drug's packaging warning of potential dangers associated with taking it.[242]

In this context, it is worth emphasising that the early part of the prosecution's narrative focused on polyneuritis, with the latter part of the document focusing on malformations in babies. This fits in well with the chronology of the unfolding of the tragedy, of course. After all, credible reports of the connection between taking thalidomide and nerve damage had come to the company by 1959 at the latest, whereas the probable connection to malformations was fully established by early 1961 at the very latest. But this focus also corresponded to the prosecution's strategy in the way they wished to argue the case: in the trial, prosecutors asked the judges to allow them to present the polyneuritis aspects of the case before presenting the evidence regarding malformations in babies, which the judges then allowed. The idea here was that the causal connection between the drug and the incidence of polyneuritis would be more easily established than the more complex connections involving malformation.[243]

The evidence was in place, the outline of the prosecution's case sketched out in the indictment and everything was ready to go. Further legal wrangling, however, led to even more delays, as did the need for extensive preparations to handle what was to be an extraordinary media event. As a result, the trial did not start until more than 15 months after the indictment was filed. In the meantime, the number of defendants actually standing before the court diminished to just seven of the nine defendants named in the indictment. Hermann Wirtz and Heinz Wolfgang Kelling were excused from taking part in the main trial on grounds of ill health.[244] A separate set of proceedings was set in train for these two, and they were later joined by a third defendant who also was excused from the main proceedings in favour of a separate trial, Dr. Gotthold-Erich Werner.[245]

Chemie Grünenthal executives on trial

When the main trial opened on 27 May 1968, it was every bit as frenzied as expected. The largest courtroom in Aachen was deemed too

242 Der leitende Oberstaatsanwalt bei dem Landgericht Aachen, 'Anklage gegen Wirtz u.a., Contergan-Verfahren'. passim.

243 Henning Sjöström, Robert Nilsson, *Thalidomide and the power of the drug companies,* p. 215.

244 'Prozesse: Contergan: Chiffre K17,' *Der Spiegel,* nr. 23/1968, pp. 47-48.

245 On the defendants and their attorneys as well as the prosecution and survivors' legal representatives, Dagmar and Karl-Heinz Wenzel, *Der Contergan-Prozess* vol. 1, pp. v-vi.

small to accommodate the combination of reporters from the international media, the lawyers and staffers on both side of the aisle and an expected large audience of interested onlookers, so it was held instead in nearby Alsdorf in the large employees' dining room (called a 'Casino' in German) of a local coal mine, the 'Anna' Grube. Each of the seven defendants at the trial was represented by at least two lawyers (Heinrich Mückter had four),[246] and they were faced on the other side of the aisle by three prosecutors and up to seven legal representatives of the 300 joint plaintiffs (i.e. the thalidomide survivors in Germany and their families). The asymmetry of resources between defence and prosecution was therefore fully evident from the start and would continue throughout the proceedings. In addition, about 100 members of the public attended each day, and about 200 journalists sat in as well, along with an endless string of witnesses and experts for both sides. It was the largest criminal trial in the history of German justice, and was expected at the outset to last one to two years.[247] When all was said and done, of course, it ended up lasting closer to three.

As mentioned, the trial has been well described, for instance in a concise overview chapter of it in Henning Sjöström and Robert Nilsson's classic *Thalidomide and the power of the drug companies,*[248] so we will not dwell on it here. But it is essential to highlight a few things, several of them every bit as bizarre as the thalidomide creation myth and other stories we have encountered in earlier chapters. Before we come to the peculiarities, however, it is worth noting again that following several days at the beginning of proceedings hammering out procedural issues, the prosecution succeeded in its request to present the polyneuritis aspects of the case first, to be followed by its presentation of the case regarding the more complex dimensions that involved malformations. As mentioned already, the complexity of the latter was perhaps a good reason for moving forward in this fashion. But it is also true that the connection between thalidomide and severe birth defects and malformations is a much more emotive, visceral issue than that between thalidomide and polyneuritis, and it therefore may have been wiser and more effective had the prosecution sought to establish the connection to malformations first. Certainly, the order of battle chosen

[246] Dagmar and Karl-Heinz Wenzel, *Der Contergan-Prozess* vol. 6, p. 8. A further defendant, Jacob Chauvistré, died in late August 1970, during the course of the trial.
[247] 'Prozesse: Contergan: Chiffre K17', *Der Spiegel,* nr. 23/1968, p. 48.
[248] See Chapter 12 of their book.

by the prosecution was considered by some to be a problem in the other large post-war criminal trial of German chemical executives, the Nuremberg IG Farben case of 1947-1948. As a member of the prosecution staff argued to chief prosecutor Josiah DuBois as that trial was just starting, 'We should have started with Auschwitz on the first day,'[249] instead of leaving this complex and emotive issue until relatively late in the proceedings.

Still, even though the prosecution presented the less startling and affective aspects of its overall case first by highlighting the tangible effects on adults affected by polyneuritis, the evidence prosecutors put forward was compelling throughout. Witnesses for, and the evidence put forward by, the prosecution were authoritative and convincing by any reasonable yardstick, but defence attorneys tried to counteract the tide of evidence favouring the prosecution's case by browbeating witnesses or by making false claims. One striking example involved their suggestion to Widukind Lenz, the physician who had played a key role in compiling the evidence about thalidomide-caused birth defects that led to its withdrawal from sale, that malformations may have been caused by an unknown virus. Lenz scoffed, pointing out that this was 'absurd'; he pointed out that there were no cases of thalidomide-like malformations in East Germany, where thalidomide had never been approved for use, and he went on to say that it was a scientific fact that even the Berlin Wall could not contain viruses. He was admonished by the judges for his understandable, if cheeky, dismissal of the defence suggestion.[250]

This exchange with Lenz and the reaction of the judges provides a good example of the fact that however absurd and obstructive the defence attorneys' tactics were, they proved surprisingly effective, although there were times when evidence presented was so damning and bizarre that even defence counsel chose not to dwell on it. One of the most striking examples involved testimony by Dr. Hilmar von Veltheim, one of Chemie Grünenthal's legal counsels, who was asked what had happened to the records of the results of tests on thalidomide conducted by the firm before the drug went to the market. He claimed that Heinrich Mückter had told him that they had been lost in the course of a move from an old to a new building; he also testified that it was impossible that the records were still in the old building. Herbert

[249] Quoted in Borkin, *The crime and punishment of IG Farben,* p. 178.
[250] Henning Sjöström, Robert Nilsson, *Thalidomide and the power of the drug companies,* p. 225.

Keller, one of the co-inventors of the drug, testified furthermore that he had no records of the experiments either, having made no copies, not only because he had not seen any use for them, but also because he was contractually bound not to use them outside of the firm.[251] The insistence that no records of experiments by the firm existed any longer was and is simply not credible, but of course very convenient for the defence's case.

The second major example of a bizarre twist to the proceedings came in conjunction with the expert testimony of Lenz, who first appeared on the stand on 12 August 1968, day 27 of the proceedings, which was also the first time the issue of malformations owing to thalidomide was touched upon.[252] In spite of repeated browbeating by the defence, which, just as in the case of the 'virus' claim we have already encountered, was allowed for the most part by Peter Weber, the lead judge in the courtroom, Lenz calmly and thoroughly testified about the ways in which he had established a causal link between thalidomide intake by pregnant women and more or less severe malformations in their babies. Unable to defeat Lenz by bullying tactics or counter-argument, defence counsel petitioned for his testimony to be disallowed, arguing that he was a biased witness and therefore could not qualify as an expert. The petition was not granted initially, but the new lead judge, Dr. Benno Dietz, who replaced Peter Weber on 9 October 1969 after he resigned owing to ill health, allowed the petition the day after he took charge of the court. Lenz's testimony was therefore formally removed from further consideration in the trial, but the grounds for this were very strange and also do not really stand up to scrutiny. Dietz insisted that this removal of Lenz's evidence from consideration did not represent a questioning of his scientific ability or credentials, and furthermore that he was not claiming that Lenz really was biased, but rather only that the defence had reasonable grounds for questioning his objectivity.[253] Exclusion of Lenz's testimony, moreover, stood in stark

[251] Dagmar and Karl-Heinz Wenzel, *Der Contergan-Prozess* vol. 2, pp. 79-80 (Veltheim), 60 (Keller). Von Veltheim's account is very similar to a story told by Mückter to an associate at Astra, the Swedish licensee of the drug. See Henning Sjöström, Robert Nilsson, *Thalidomide and the power of the drug companies,* pp. 188-189, 230-233.

[252] Lenz's testimony from day 27 to day 42 of the trial is summarised in Dagmar and Karl-Heinz Wenzel, *Der Contergan-Prozess* vol. 1, pp. 172-238. Note that day 27 of the trial occurred many weeks after the trial began because the day number referred only to days on which proceedings took place, i.e. not on weekend days or during holidays or recesses.

[253] Henning Sjöström, Robert Nilsson, *Thalidomide and the power of the drug companies,* pp. 223-226, 249, 252.

contrast to the willingness of the court (and the prosecution) to accept the testimony of expert witnesses who were close to Chemie Grüenthal (and therefore clearly partial) such as Werner Schulemann.

The third major oddity involved the actual abandonment of the trial on 18 December 1970. The judges made it clear that they did not consider the defendants innocent, and we will go into some of the reasons they put forward for this view later in the chapter. Here, what is important to emphasise is that the judges considered that because the defendants' 'guilt was relatively limited' and because there was 'no public interest' in continuing the trial, it should be discontinued. There had been to that point 283 days of proceedings over the course of well over two and a half years.[254] The judges' written opinion explaining the decision to suspend the trial listed a number of mitigating circumstances for the defendants that militated towards ending proceedings, one of which was that a 'legally binding' offer of compensation for thalidomide survivors from Chemie Grünenthal was on the table.[255]

At first glance, the existence of this offer might make the trial's suspension seem a perfectly reasonable way of proceeding. But the oddity here is this: *it is not possible to have an out-of-court settlement in a criminal trial,*[256] which is effectively what this settlement offer entailed.

So, how did this happen? A number of important questions arise from this general one:

- How and why did the federal government decide to contribute about half of the total sum of the settlement?
- Why did Chemie Grünenthal agree to pay for the (very considerable) costs of the trial when the normal procedure in case of such an abandonment of proceedings by the prosecution was for the state to bear the costs?[257]

[254] Dagmar and Karl-Heinz Wenzel, *Der Contergan-Prozess* vol. 6, pp. 7-8.

[255] Medizinisch Pharmazeutische Studiengesellschaft e.V., Dokumentation III/71, 'Schriftlicher Einstellungsbeschluß der Ersten Großen Strafkammer des Landgerichts Aachen im sog. Contergan-Verfahren', Frankfurt, 1971, pp. 70-74. Quotation from p.74.

[256] This became possible later in specific circumstances under a subsequent modification of the same paragraph of the German legal code (paragraph 153) that was used to suspend this trial. See for instance Christian Sylt, 'The real reason Bernie Ecclestone settled his bribery trial,' *Forbes* (20 August 2014), available at: *http://www.forbes.com/sites/csylt/2014/08/20/therealreasonbernieecclestonesettledhisbriberytrial/#2b6e1bef5020* <viewed 14 July 2016>. But it was not permissible at the time of the trial of Chemie Grünenthal executives, and the public outcry at the settlement of the Ecclestone trial would certainly have been much greater in the case of the thalidomide trial had this explicit connection been made.

[257] Dagmar and Karl-Heinz Wenzel, *Der Contergan-Prozess* vol. 6, p. 8.

- And, most importantly, how exactly did the court decide to suspend criminal proceedings in return for what was in effect an out-of-court settlement?

We will try to answer these questions in the next section of this chapter, but, put briefly, the process by which the abandonment came about started not all that long after the trial began and was prompted by the Wirtz family, who owned Chemie Grünenthal, and their lawyers. The suspension itself resulted from extensive negotiations between the company, the federal government and a number of other parties, although crucially they did not include the families of thalidomide-damaged children or their legal representatives until most of the details had already been worked out. These negotiations therefore affected the trial's outcome, and they did so through means that were at best shady and in the legal twilight, if not downright illegal and unconstitutional. And the ultimate outcome was the establishment of a foundation that those who created it – not to mention those who 'benefitted' from it – knew was underfunded and inadequate from the start.

Constructing a way out: Preparing to end the trial

The trial of executives of Chemie Grünenthal started on 27 May 1968. Just over thirteen months later, the Wirtz family, the owners of the company (and one of whom, of course, had been charged in the indictment and was standing trial), began to implement a strategy that would eventually stop it. Mobilising their lawyers, Dr. Günter Dörr and Frank Dahrendorf, both of whom were active in the ongoing trial in Alsdorf, along with the Wirtz family's considerable connections in government, they were able to arrange a meeting between Wirtz family members, accompanied by their lawyers, and personnel from the Federal Ministry for Health on 3 July 1969 'to discuss questions that could arise in connection with the winding up [Abwicklung] of the Contergan trial'. The meeting started with a presentation from the Chemie Grünenthal side. The firm was considering making 'a considerable sum' available for 'the mitigation of the injuries ... that had been sustained by the joint plaintiffs who were represented in the Contergan trial'. And, although those representing the company claimed that they expected a 'not guilty' verdict, they stated that they wished 'to do something out of court [außergerichtlich] to improve the fate of the children affected'.[258]

So far, so good. However, the Health Ministry officials undoubtedly knew a 'but' was coming, and they did not have long to wait. The stumbling block for Grünenthal revolved around the issue of how to come up with a settlement that dealt with all of the claims of the children concerned without innumerable civil lawsuits that would be 'stressful and costly for all of those involved'. The funds spent on such trials, the firm's representatives continued, would be 'better channelled to the affected parties directly following an out-of-court agreement'. In the discussion that immediately followed, all of those present agreed that it would be necessary, if also very difficult, for all of the providers of social security and welfare (who were already providing social and medical services to thalidomide providers and therefore would have to be on board) to come to 'an out-of-court agreement', and, furthermore, that if this did not work out it would probably only be possible to achieve 'a settlement ... through a government regulation [Vorschrift] that would apply to all concerned [mit Wirkung gegenüber Allen]'. The discussion continued: 'A legal regulation along these lines was not ruled out entirely, but the difficulties were certainly extraordinarily large.'[259]

At the end of the meeting, the representatives of Grünenthal asked the Ministry of Health to check with all bodies responsible for social insurance and social aid to see if it would be possible to realise a general agreement that would solve all of the claims arising from the thalidomide (Contergan) trial at once. The final word fell to the head of Section I (Abteilung I) of the Health Ministry: he 'indicated that the Foundation for the Disabled Child [Stiftung für das behinderte Kind]

[258] BMGes Referat I B 1, 'Betr.: Contergan-Verfahren; hier: Besuch der leitenden Herren des Contergan-Herstellerwerkes am 3. Juli 1969 in BMGes', 21 July 1969, in BArch B 189/751, Bl. 5-6, quotations Bl. 5. Although the document indicates the presence of the 'Gebruder Wirtz', Niklas Lenhard-Schramm in 'Die Haltung; (p. 28) makes the well taken point that this could not refer to Hermann Wirtz (who was being prosecuted) and one or more of his brothers since at that time his two brothers were both deceased. Lenhard-Schramm, however, draws the conclusion from this that the document could not possibly be referring to Hermann Wirtz, which does not follow: it could refer to Hermann Wirtz as representative of the Wirtz brothers firm, or to Hermann Wirtz and another member of his family, perhaps his son, Michael. Regardless, the key point here is this, and it is undisputable: *a member or members of the Wirtz family and the lawyers who were representing them and their fellow defendants in the Alsdorf trial met while the criminal trial was still underway with officials in the Federal Ministry of Health to try to arrange an end to that trial by means of a cash settlement.*

[259] BMGes Referat I B 1, 'Betr.: Contergan-Verfahren; hier: Besuch der leitenden Herren des Contergan-Herstellerwerkes am 3. Juli 1969 in BMGes', 21 July 1969, in BArch B 189/751, Bl. 5-6.

appeared to be suitable for the practical implementation of the settlement of claims'.[260]

It is worth pausing to consider the context and significance of this meeting because it set out many of the key issues that would be involved in, and possible ways forward to, ending the trial.

First, it is important that the two lawyers attending the meeting had been involved in a public relations effort to raise hopes about a settlement. Dörr had indicated in a press conference at the end of April 1969 that the firm was in serious discussion with representatives of the parents concerned about a settlement, while Dahrendorf refused to comment on a press report that the sum under discussion was DM 150 million[261] (even though the most likely source of this reported figure was Grünenthal itself, which had set up a press office to 'inform' reporters at the trial).[262] So, one of the key points emerging already by mid-1969 was the idea of a settlement along with an order of magnitude for the sum involved.

The second point was that this would be an out-of-court settlement which was clearly connected to ending the trial (and ensuring that there would be no further liability for Chemie Grünenthal) even though at this point the representatives of the firm were at pains to indicate that they did not expect a guilty verdict and that there was no explicit causal connection established yet between the trial's outcome and the settlement.

The third key issue involved the veiled threat that the sum that would be available for a settlement would be whittled away by legal action unless some sort of overall agreement were reached.

Fourth, it was clear already from this July meeting that discussions about how to come to an agreement would involve negotiations among a large number of parties, but it is important to underscore that *the affected families were not mentioned as being part of the discussions.*

Fifth, the idea was introduced that the only way to gain an overall agreement would be through legislation or through imposing government regulations, something that would pose 'extraordinarily large' difficulties to enact, but which already appeared to be the only game in town.

260 *Ibid.,* Bl. 6-7. The German version of this quotation is: 'Abteilungsleiter I wies darauf hin, daß für die praktische Durchführung der Schadensregulierung die Stiftung für das behinderte Kind geeignet erscheine.'

261 Henning Sjöström, Robert Nilsson, *Thalidomide and the power of the drug companies,* p. 245.

262 *Ibid.,* p. 213.

Sixth, although not stated explicitly at this meeting in July 1969, it was implicit (and soon made explicit) that the firm would only agree to a settlement which would involve no admission of guilt and no additional liabilities for any future claims.

A final point needs to be highlighted regarding this meeting of July 1969. Although it is not clear whether the idea of using the Foundation for the Disabled Child as a vehicle 'suitable for the practical implementation of the settlement of claims'[263] came from the firm and its representatives or from the officials of the Ministry of Health, this statement indicates unequivocally that the notion of channelling funds through a third-party body that would be at arm's length from both the firm and the federal government was floated quite early in the negotiations that would eventually lead to the end of the trial in return for payment of a settlement. In this case, the foundation mentioned was a privately funded one that had been set up not long before, in June 1967, primarily to ensure that the survivors of the thalidomide disaster received 'direct and unbureaucratic support', although with a remit that also included provision of aid for children whose physical or mental disabilities had other causes.[264] By late September 1969, the idea of using this particular foundation as a conduit to dispense the firm's compensation to thalidomide survivors had been discarded, although, as we shall see later in the chapter, some of the earlier thinking continued: an attorney representing Chemie Grünenthal presented a suggested way forward in October 1969 that involved not only a charitable foundation, but also one that would provide aid to all disabled children, and not just those who had been damaged by thalidomide.[265]

During the weeks that followed, representatives of the Federal Health Ministry liaised intensively with their counterparts in other federal ministries, including the Ministry of Labour (BMA) and the Interior Ministry (BMI), although they deliberately kept the Ministries

[263] BMGes Referat I B 1, 'Betr.: Contergan-Verfahren; hier: Besuch der leitenden Herren des Contergan-Herstellerwerkes am 3. Juli 1969 in BMGes', 21 July 1969, in BArch B 189/751, Bl. 6-7. The German version of this quotation is: 'Abteilungsleiter I wies darauf hin, daß für die praktische Durchführung der Schadensregulierung die Stiftung für das behinderte Kind geeignet erscheine.'

[264] 'Die Geschichte der Stiftung für das behinderte Kind', available at: *http://www.stiftung-behindertes-kind.de/stiftung/geschichte.html* <viewed 22 September 2016>.

[265] Lenhard-Schramm, 'Die Haltung', p. 626. The attorney's suggestion (Frank Dahrendorf, Betr. Ueberlegungen zur Situation der behinderten Kinder in der Bundesrepublik Deutschland, 6 October 1969, BArch B 122/10839, Bl. 372-377) is examined in detail later in this chapter.

of Economics and Finance out of the loop because of an undertaking to Chemie Grünenthal to keep the whole matter confidential. Reporting on progress in these discussions in a memo to his Health Ministry section leader dated 18 September 1969, Mr. Harsdorf (Referent I B 1) noted a number of obstacles to a solution along the lines sketched out in July that had been raised in talks with other Ministries. Again, part of the issue involved precedent. The Interior Ministry stressed that the participation of the federal government in an overall settlement could lead to pressure on the government to put taxpayer money towards hardship funds to compensate survivors. The Interior and Health Ministries furthermore expressed 'considerable reservations' about 'an engagement of the federal government', especially because this would lead eventually to the matter having to be taken up at the 'political level'. For its part, the Labour Ministry (BMA) was also anxious about establishing possible precedents, in particular if a large number of claimants came forward, but also in the event of another medical disaster of this sort. BMA representatives, however, wanted to expand the range of participation in talks to develop a settlement by bringing in 'representatives of groups [Kreisen] of those affected', in other words including the families of thalidomide children. With regard to this latter suggestion, Harsdorf quickly interrupted to ask for a decision on the inclusion of representatives of the thalidomiders and their families in negotiations to be postponed pending approval from a 'higher level'. His section leader apparently agreed; there was a large handwritten exclamation point next to the report's mention of the BMA's suggestion.[266] Clearly there was no great appetite at this point on the part of the civil service to muddy the waters with inputs from the families of those injured by the drug or their representatives.

The final paragraph of Harsdorf's memo, however, was the most telling. First of all, he drew the following conclusion from the talks held with other ministries to date: dealing with the idea of an overall settlement, possibly brokered through the federal government, would require input from a number of different governmental and non-governmental bodies, which meant that there would be no way to keep the matter confidential. This in turn would entail violating the conditions that had been agreed earlier with the company. More importantly and tellingly, however, he also noted that there was a real

266 BMGes (Harsdorf, Referent IB1), Memo, 18 September 1969, BArch B 189/751, Bl. 13-15.

possibility that this sort of broad discussion of, and decision on, an overall settlement might raise the impression that it was directly and causally linked to the end of the trial. Harsdorf concluded with a recommendation to his superiors (remember, the memo was meant for his section leader, who would presumably have taken the suggestion up with those higher up still in the ministry):

> *For these reasons, it seems advisable ... to enter into discussions on the solution to the problem only when the trial is finished because then, too, an influence over the trial need not be feared when news of the negotiations becomes known to the public.*[267]

Harsdorf's advice was very sensible: there should be no possible public perception of a causal connection between the end of the trial and the agreement of a settlement, which would be insured if the former were ended before negotiations on the latter started. But his sound counsel was already in the process of being completely ignored. During autumn and winter 1969/1970, and culminating at the beginning of spring 1970, the German federal government helped broker a deal that ensured that the trial would be discontinued in return for a settlement for the children affected by thalidomide, one which was extremely disadvantageous to the survivors of the thalidomide catastrophe and which, at the same time, protected Chemie Grünenthal, the company that had wreaked this havoc. Crucially, the explicit connection between the settlement and the end of the trial was not mentioned publicly, not only because of aversion to public reaction, but also because this could have led to investigation of the legality and/or constitutionality of all of this. Not for the first – or last – time in history, a government intervened to preserve the interests of a small number of executives of a powerful company rather than those of the large number of people damaged by their actions.

Although it would be possible, on the basis of a large number of official documents that we have collected and analysed, to produce a detailed, blow-by-blow chronology of the process by which this settlement emerged, that would run the risk of losing the most important general points in the factual detail.[268] Instead, we focus

[267] *Ibid.*, Bl. 15.

[268] A detailed, blow-by-blow chronology summarising a very large number of archival documents is available in Lenhard-Schramm, 'Die Haltung', especially Chapter 3, section 3.4.

thematically on four key aspects of the process by which the trial was ended in return for payment of a settlement:

- Who was involved and in what ways?
- How was the final sum of the settlement arrived at?
- What form would the settlement take?
- And, crucially, what was the exact connection between the agreement of the settlement and the end of the trial?

WHO WAS INVOLVED?

The cast of the drama that would culminate in an initial settlement of claims of thalidomide victims in return for ending the trial was large. But it is important to underscore at the outset who was *not* involved, at least until after the major contours of the agreement had been determined. The parents of the children affected by thalidomide and their legal representatives had *no input whatsoever* into the detailed negotiations undertaken by the other parties (whom we will come to shortly) during late 1969 and the first ten weeks of 1970 that culminated in draft legislation. In fact, as late as 10 March 1970, in a response to a request from a representative of the Association of People Damaged by Contergan to see the draft as it stood at that point, the Federal Minister of Justice stated explicitly that he would not under any circumstances 'at this stage in the negotiations' permit 'the Association to receive this paper from us already at this time'.[269] The parents' legal representatives were only brought into the fold and provided with the draft legislation and information on the proposed foundation that would administer the settlement on 16 March 1970, and they explicitly registered their 'regret' at this state of affairs at the start of their meeting on that day with officials from the Ministries of Justice, Work and Health.[270]

[269] Pers. Referentin, *BMJ*, Vermerk für Herrn Diller, 10 March 1970, BArch B141/59478, Bl. 149.
[270] Memo (BMGes), Betr.: Stiftung 'Hilfswerk für das behinderte Kind', 17 March 1970, BArch B141/59479, Bl. 5-8. This is a key point overlooked by Lenhard-Schramm in 'Die Haltung': in spite of his repeated insistence that all parties were involved in negotiations to end the trial from the outset, he himself admits that the draft legislation from 2 March 1970 that was laid before the families and their representatives on 16 March 'machte den Vergleichsvertrag vom 10. April [between Chemie Grünenthal and the families in relation to compensation for the thalidomide disaster] obsolet..., bevor dieser überhaupt abgeschlossen wurde...' (p. 630) Essentially, then, the families were kept away from the negotiations between the firm and representatives of state and local government until the latter had reached preliminary agreement. Otherwise they would not have been surprised and disappointed at seeing it for the first time only in mid-March.

So, who came up with the draft legislation and the other details? At the centre of those who were involved in the process were officials from the Federal Ministry of Health, who kicked off coordinated discussions with other federal ministries following the visit from Wirtz family members and their legal representatives in early July 1969, along with the Federal Ministry of Justice. Crucially, the Federal Justice Ministry was also in close contact with the state secretary in the North Rhine Westphalian Ministry of Justice, Baron von Münchhausen, who provided a direct link to his superior, Justice Minister Josef Neuberger, and also a direct conduit to the prosecutor's office in Aachen.[271]

But there was also intervention from another quarter in Bonn at a 'higher level'. Federal President Gustav Heinemann – who had been associated with the thalidomide catastrophe earlier in his capacity as attrorney for a Chemie Grünenthal manager whom prosecutors decided not to put on trial[272] – and personnel from his office became closely involved in the negotiations and influenced the ultimate outcome, which again involved contact with Chemie Grünenthal's legal representatives, but also with Baron von Münchhausen and with federal government ministries.[273] Heinemann, however, was also involved in bringing others into the fray, including representatives of the chemical industry[274] as well as prominent representatives of what we would now call the 'third sector', including churches and charities, specifically the Archbishop of Cologne, Joseph Cardinal Höffner; the President of the Lutheran Church in the Rhineland, Professor D. Joachim Bochmann; and the

271 BMGes Referat I B 1, 'Betr.: Contergan-Verfahren; hier: Besuch der leitenden Herren des Contergan-Herstellerwerkes am 3. Juli 1969 in BMGes', 21 July 1969, BArch B 189/751, Bl. 5-6; Secretary of State, Federal Ministry of Justice, Memorandum Betr. Contergan, 11 March 1970, BArch B 141/59478/152-153.

272 See correspondence between Gustav Heinemann and Dr. Günther Nowel from May 1963, in *Archiv der sozialen Demokratie,* Bonn, Nachlass Gustav W. Heinemann, Teil 2, Nr. 01476.

273 Various documents on this from late 1969 and early 1970 are in BArch B 122/10839. See also Münchhausen (Federal Ministry of Justice, North Rhine Westphalia) to Regierungsdirektor Buhrow (Bundespräsidialamt), Betr. Contergan-Verfahren, 27 January 1970, BArch B 141/59477, Bl. 10-11. The fact that a copy of this letter is in the archival record group consisting of files of the Federal Ministry of Justice is an indication of how closely the President's Office kept in touch with federal government ministries.

274 Horst Ehmke (Bundeskanzleramt) to Gustav Heinemann, 5 January 1970 (personal and confidential), BArch B 122/. Ehmke suggested that if the amount that can be brought to bear by Chemie Grünenthal for the settlement were not enough, the 'whole chemical industry in solidarity' could make up the difference. Here, we have a connection between the president's Office and the chancellor of the Federal Republic through Ehmke, who was on 'Du' terms with the president.

Chair of the Aktion Sorgekind foundation, Lotte Lemke.[275] The purpose of all of this, it needs to be stressed, was not only to mobilise influential people to campaign to settle all outstanding claims against Chemie Grünenthal, but also to raise additional funds for that purpose from industry and the third sector.

We will come back to the funding arrangements very shortly. Here, it is necessary to note one more participant in the negotiation process, Horst Pelckmann, who managed to gain access to the President's Office for this purpose after taking up contact in late November 1969 with the wife of the President's secretary of state, Diether Spangenberger. Pelckmann, who had had a long career in the German Foreign Service, latterly in the United States, until he retired in December 1969, represents a figure in the shadows of this drama. It is not entirely clear why he was so interested in the matter (he repeatedly underscored that he had no connection to any of the parties concerned), nor why he was taken so seriously. But he was; Pelckmann appeared regularly at meetings in the President's Office and gave important – and telling – legal advice about the way in which the eventual settlement could be implemented.[276] Before we look at that advice, though, we need to examine the way in which the amount of the settlement was determined and who would contribute to it.

How much should the settlement be, and who should pay?

Pretty much from the outset of negotiations, the sum Chemie Grünenthal was willing to contribute towards a settlement amounted to DM 100 million, and that is in the end what was on offer, although a few small additional concessions were made along the way. Was that sum enough?

The parents of the thalidomiders and their legal representatives did not think so. They estimated that a figure that might cover the total damages adequately would be something in the range of DM 1.5 billion, and, without explicitly agreeing to that higher amount, a civil

[275] Bundespräsident pers. Referent (Buhrow) to Beckmann, Höffner, and Lemke, 6 December 1969 (confidential), BArch B 122/10389, Bl. 357-359. The letter refers to a meeting that had taken place in the President's Office with the three addressees on 5 November 1960.

[276] Various documents by or about Pelckmann from late 1969 and early 1970 are in BArch B 122/10839. See in particular Pelckmann to Frau Gisele Spangenberger (Roy Blumenthal International Associates Inc., Berlin), 30 November 1969, in this file, Bl. 365, and attachments, which included a memo on the case, his interest in it, and some advice (Bl. 366-367) and his CV, Bl. 368.

servant in the federal government admitted that, 'The sum of 100 million DM is ... insufficient to do justice to the needs of the Contergan children to a reasonable extent.'[277] A response by Bahlmann in the Justice Ministry to a set of queries from Buhrow in the President's Office a little earlier, in late 1969, was more frank, however, indicating that 'the sum that has been mentioned for compensation stands in no relationship to the damages, which are estimated to be in the billions'.[278] In other words, even government officials indicated in official correspondence that the families' estimate of DM 1.5 billion was probably, if anything, far too low. Implicitly, then, the firm's offer of around DM 100 million was derisory.

Regardless of this, though, it is of course clear why Chemie Grünenthal might wish to stick to the very, very low figure that it had placed on the table. What is less clear is whether the firm might have been able to afford a lot more. Indeed, the Federal Ministry of Justice posed a question exactly along these lines to federal government auditors around the end of 1969: 'Is 100 million DM the upper limit of what might be economically reasonable [for the firm] ... or where does this limit lie?'[279] As far as we can tell from the documents we have seen, that question was never answered directly, although Baron von Münchhausen may have provided a clue as to why the government did not pursue it further in a letter to the President's Office from late January 1970, writing that '...it has been told to me in confidence that this matter [i.e. the settlement] is not just urgent for those damaged. It is even more urgent also because the financial strength of Chemie Grünenthal is recognisably and considerably on the downturn.'[280]

Whether or not Chemie Grünenthal could afford to pay more than DM 100 million, however, even if the financial circumstances of the firm were as bad in reality as von Münchhausen hinted in early 1970, it was unlikely to affect its ability to pay out, as indicated in an expert report prepared by the North Rhine Westphalian Justice Ministry in spring 1969 about the mechanisms for bringing proceedings to a close through suspension. At that time, the Ministry judged the idea that

[277] [Author unknown], 'Begründung', n.d. [mid-late 1969], BArch B189/751, Bl. 80.

[278] Bahlmann (FMJ – Bundesministerium fuer Justiz, the Federal Ministry for Justice) to Buhrow (President's Office), 18 December 1969, BArch B 122/10839, Bl. 331-332, quotation Bl. 332.

[279] State secretary FMJ, Vermerk: Betr. Contergan (handmarked: Eilt), 17 March 1970, BArch B 141/59479, Bl. 3.

[280] Münchhausen to Buhrow, 27 January 1970 (personal), BArch B 141/59477, Bl. 10-11, quotation Bl. 11.

Chemie Grünenthal would go into receivership before being able to pay out to the children to be 'unlikely'. What is more, and this point applied to early 1970 as well, even if that unlikely event were to come to pass, the survivors would be able to make civil claims again the 'Dalli – Maurer & Wirtz firm (in addition to subsidiaries)'.[281]

Nevertheless, if one assumes that most German authorities bought into the notion that DM 100 million was the upper limit of what the firm could afford – and they seem to have done so, by and large – the only options were either to encourage acceptance of the offer or to try to top it up in some way or another, perhaps through funds supplied by the federal government, perhaps from other sources. Here, the approaches by the Federal President's Office to the chemical and pharmaceutical industries and the churches mentioned above formed part of this effort to get additional funding, but success was limited. For its part, the chemical industry representatives declared themselves willing to contribute, but not if the foundation were limited exclusively to support for the children damaged by thalidomide, and the same was true of the pharmaceutical industry. This idea of a more generalised foundation for all children with disabilities was one that continued for some time, forming the basis of much of the negotiations among federal ministries and involving Chemie Grünenthal (but not representatives of the children affected) during the first ten weeks of 1970. The churches, on the other hand, viewed their role in the ultimate settlement differently from the way the government might have wished. According to an internal report in the Federal Justice Ministry of a conversation with the head of the Catholic bureau in Bonn initiated by Dr. von Weiszäcker, a member of the Bundestag, the idea of putting up DM 100 million towards the foundation was, for the churches, 'utopian'. The report continued, indicating that, 'The churches view their task as lying ... not in direct financial compensation for the Contergan children, but rather in providing support [einer Förderung] for the ... facilities' to be created to administer the work of the foundation after its establishment.[282]

281 Expert report of the North Rhine Westphalian Justice Ministry, n.d. [ca. Spring 1969], LA NRW Duisburg, Ger Rep 0139 00363, Bl. 0091-0096, quotation from Bl. 0091.

282 On the idea of additional support from the federal government, industry, or the churches, Abteilungsleiter S, Memo for attention of State Secretary Manger-Koenig, Betr. Contergan-Schäden, 9 March 1970, BArch B 189/156718. This document also indicates the willingness of the chemical industry to contribute under the condition that the beneficiaries of the foundation not be restricted to thalidomide victims, while the pharmaceutical industry trade association later made the same in its representations to federal government officials. See Vermerk Betr.:

In the end, for reasons that are not entirely clear from the documents we have been able to locate, the ultimate decision was for Chemie Grünenthal to put up DM 100 million as originally envisaged. This sum was, in addition, in the end enhanced to some small degree by virtue of the fact that administrative costs of the foundation would be paid by Chemie Grünenthal, and there was also a fund set up for the victims of thalidomide-induced polyneuritis. The firm also assumed the costs of the trial,[283] something that was extremely unusual in the case of suspended proceedings, where the state usually pays all costs. This was quite probably in exchange for an eventual federal government contribution towards the foundation, which was originally envisaged to be between DM 50-100 million.

Even with the government top-up (which ended up being DM 110 million, although only DM 50 million of that was earmarked specifically for survivors of thalidomide), however, the settlement was paltry. And, to add insult to injury, the firm's main contribution proved in the end to be even smaller in real terms than even the miserly top-line figure indicated. Astonishingly, a 1976 expert report prepared by the Federal Ministry of Justice estimated that, owing to various tax savings resulting from write-offs that the company could claim as a result of its contribution, 'the effective economic burden on the GmbH [Chemie Grünenthal] amounted to between DM 35.7 and 29.4 million'. In other words, the 'burden' of the settlement on the firm in real terms was just a third of the company's nominal contribution![284]

There can be no question then: the firm got off practically scot-free, and its managers got off the hook for their role in the crime that had taken place; the federal government was deeply involved; and those who had suffered the worst effects of thalidomide were victimised once again, this time by virtue of a completely inadequate settlement the

Entwurf eines Gesetzes zur Rerrichtung einer nationalen Stiftung 'Hilfswerk für das behinderte Kind,' 1 July 1970, BArch B 141/59481, Bl. 159. For continued discussions about the possibility of such a non-exclusive foundation, Referat III/I, Vermerk Betr. Nationalstiftung für behinderte Kinder, 10 February 1970, BArch B 122/10839, Bl. 303. For the report on the churches' position, FMJ Ref. IVA (MDgt Diller), Report, Betr.: Stiftung 'Hilfswerk für das behinderte Kind', 10 March 1970, BArch B 141/59478, Bl.171-172 (quotation from 172).

283 Dagmar and Karl-Heinz Wenzel, *Der Contergan-Prozess* vol. 6, p. 8 (where Wenzel and Wenzel note how unusual it was for costs to be assumed by the defendants in the case of a suspension of a trial), and facsimile of letter from Wirtz and Wirtz dated 18 December 1970 offering to take over the costs and to provide compensation also to those affected by polyneuritis, pp. 268-269.

284 FMJ Referat IV B 1 (MD Ninnemann), Betr.: Stiftung 'Hilfswerk für behinderte Kinder', 15 October 1976, BArch B141/59506, Bl. 179-189; quotation from p. 8 (Bl. 186).

main contours of which had been negotiated and defined behind their backs.

What form should the settlement take?

Very quickly, and in spite of the reluctance expressed through September 1969 about a legislative solution to the issue of compensation for thalidomide victims, it became clear that just such a solution was the only game in town, as had been implicit since July 1969 when Wirtz family members and their lawyers had met to discuss this with officials from the Federal Health Ministry. Moreover, the idea of using a foundation to dispense compensation to survivors had also been aired at that meeting in July 1969. The issues to be resolved to make this happen involved the form of the legislation and the specific charitable foundation that would implement it as well as, of course, the issue of how all of this might relate to the trial. As mentioned in the previous subsection, from July 1969 at the latest there seems to have been support for the idea that the foundation should not be restricted to the victims of the thalidomide disaster, but rather that its funds should be available to all disabled children, and this notion continued as more concrete discussions took place. No doubt, the main idea here was to avoid any recognition of guilt or responsibility, especially for those companies in the chemical and pharmaceuticals industries other than Chemie Grünenthal.[285]

But, although civil servants in the federal government were instrumental in coming up with the eventual draft of legislation and the form of the foundation, two extra-governmental figures had a particularly important role in shaping them. The first was none other than Frank Dahrendorf, defence attorney at the Alsdorf trial and legal representative of the Grünenthal firm, who wrote to the Federal President's Office on 6 October 1969 with some detailed suggestions on how to proceed. He started off with some facts and statistics that had recently been published by a journalist on the number of disabled children in the Federal Republic and the types of disabilities they had, following this with some general thoughts on the responsibility of society for taking care of these children and their families. His letter then continued with a section on the idea of establishing a foundation

[285] Vermerk Betr.: Entwurf eines Gesetzes zur Rerrichtung einer nationalen Stiftung 'Hilfswerk für das behinderte Kind,' 1 July 1970, BArch B 141/59481, Bl. 159.

to do just this (which took the place of the earlier idea of funnelling the money through an existing foundation). In the final section of the document, though, he came to the point. Again, he started off with the general claim that, 'It corresponds to my political conviction that in every civilised state aid of this sort [i.e. for children with disabilities] is a duty of society.' But he then moved quickly to specific issues in this regard for the firm he represented, underscoring that a large contribution from the company could form the basis for such a fund. He ended up by stressing:

> *[On the one hand] the Chemie Grünenthal firm does not expect to save any sums [of money] by virtue of paying into an 'industry fund' or a 'national foundation'. On the other hand, it will obviously have to be certain in the case of a participation by the firm ... in a foundation of this sort that no additional financial risks in connection with the malformations that have been ascribed to thalidomide can be assigned to the company.*[286]

The argument and the suggestion were as cynical as they were effective in shaping the thinking of government officials as they proceeded further with discussions into spring 1970.

The second person outside of government who had an important impact on discussions was Horst Pelckmann, whom we encountered earlier. Again, he was not affiliated with the firm, nor was he associated with the plaintiffs. But he was clearly interested, for whatever reason, in helping develop a legislative and regulatory framework within which a settlement could be made. Here, one of the suggestions he made was as extraordinary as it was influential. It was extraordinary because it drew explicitly on the experiences of IG Farben, a company that Pelckmann was intimately familiar with, having served as counsel for one of its directors who was tried at Nuremberg in the late 1940s.[287] Pelckmann's suggestion was based on another aspect of IG Farben's post-war fate. In 1953, Frankfurt Regional Court found in favour of the plaintiff in an action against IG Farbenindustrie in Liquidation (i.L.) (the post-war

[286] Abt. II/1, Vermerk, 16 October 1969, and Frank Dahrendorf, Betr. Ueberlegungen zur Situation der behinderten Kinder in der Bundesrepublik Deutschland, 6 October 1969, BArch B 122/10839, Bl. 371, 372-377 respectively, quotation Bl. 377.

[287] On Pelckmann as defence attorney for August von Knierheim, who had been a member of the IG Farben managing board as well as its chief counsel, see Kim Christian Priemel, *The Betrayal: The Nuremberg Trials and German Divergence* (Oxford: Oxford University Press, 2016) pp. 229-230.

legal successor to the IG Farben chemical firm), former concentration camp inmate Norbert Wollheim. Wollheim had worked for IG Farben's Auschwitz plant as a forced labourer. IG Farben i.L. was found culpable for violating Wollheim's rights, and the court therefore ordered that compensation be paid. The company promptly appealed, but the combination of uncertainty of success in its appeal along with absolute certainty that many other plaintiffs would soon follow Wollheim's example prompted the company to seek another solution. The German government obliged with the IG Farben Notice to Creditors Act, passed on 19 April 1957 with effect from 27 May. It stipulated that certain claims against the firm – not surprisingly, those of forced labourers for the most part – would no longer be valid after 1 January 1958. Those who might make such claims were invited to do so by 31 December 1957, and they would then be eligible for funds that would be paid by IG Farben i.L. into, and distributed by, the Claims Conference, which had been founded in 1951 to deal with compensation claims from Jewish victims of Nazism. The total offered by the firm was DM 30 million, with 90% targeted for former forced labourers who were Jewish, and 10% for those who were not. Thereafter, IG Farben i.L. would have no further liability and would be immune from further claims.[288]

This does sound awfully familiar! Pelckmann wrote to Buhrow in the President's Office on 27 January 1970 with information on the earlier legislation, citing it as 'a precedent for the Contergan case' and as a way of dealing with the difficulty identified by the federal government of getting a single solution that would 'accommodate all remaining issues at the same time'.[289] Pelckmann's suggestion was not implemented directly, but it was highly influential nonetheless. Although, not surprisingly, the references to IG Farben soon disappeared from further documents and are not to be found in any public pronouncements, there is no question that the Notice to Creditors Act formed a precedent and even part of the basis for the eventual legislative solution passed by the Bundestag on 17 December 1971, the day before the first anniversary of the trial's suspension. The Law to Create a Foundation [Stiftung] 'Hilfswerk für behinderte Kinder' ('Aid

288 'The settlement negotiations between I.G. Farben i.L. and the Claims Conference': *http://www.wollheim-memorial.de/en/vergleichsverhandlungs_en* <viewed 25 August 2015>.

289 Pelckmann to Buhrow, 27 January 1970; Persönliches Büro, Vermerk Betr. Contergan-Prozeß, 27 January 1969; both in BArch B122/10839, Bl. 310-311 and Bl. 309 respectively. First quotation is from Bl. 310, and second from Bl. 309.

Organisation for Disabled Children')[290] took effect on 31 October 1972. Not only was its funding inadequate (as was the earlier IG Farben compensation fund), the pitiful sums involved were not even earmarked exclusively for those children damaged by thalidomide, but rather offered aid to other disabled children as well (just as the IG Farben included both Jewish and non-Jewish survivors of the company's use of slave labour in the Nazi era).

WAS THERE A CONNECTION BETWEEN THE AGREEMENT ON THE SETTLEMENT AND THE END OF THE TRIAL?

In their written decision on the suspension of the trial, the judges noted that the 'legally binding' agreement for Chemie Grünenthal to provide 'DM 110 million including interest' to surviving thalidomide-affected children was one of a number of factors that they listed in mitigation of the grave misdeeds of the defendants.[291] But here, as in other public documents produced at the time, care was exercised so as not to acknowledge any causal connection between the two events. However, although it is extremely rare in historical research to be able to establish such a causal connection without any reservations at all, in this case it is. And it is rarer still to be able to establish such a connection on the basis of a document that is a 'smoking gun', but in this case there is not just one, but rather many.

We will look at the contents of a small number of such documents shortly. The first point that needs to be made, however, is that the issue of the connection between the settlement and the end of the trial was made early on, and not only by those from the federal government and the firm who had a clear interest in establishing it. In a letter to President of the Federal Republic Gustav Heinemann, dated 28 October 1969, Joseph Cardinal Höffner, Archbishop of Cologne posed a series of questions that linked the two explicitly. To paraphrase the Archbishop:

[290] 'Gesetz über die Errichtung eienr Stiftung "Hilfswerk für behinderte Kinder"', 17 December 1971, in Bundesgesetzblatt Teil I (1971), available on-line at: *http://www.bgbl.de/xaver/bgbl/start.xav?start=%2F%2F*%5B%40attr_id%3D%27bgbl171s2018.pdf%27%5D#__bgbl__%2F%2F*%5B%40attr_id%3D%27bgbl171s2018.pdf%27%5D__1474630929256* <viewed 23 September 2016>.

[291] Medizinisch Pharmazeutische Studiengesellschaft e.V., Dokumentation III/71, 'Schriftlicher Einstellungsbeschluß der Ersten Großen Strafkammer des Landgerichts Aachen im sog. Contergan-Verfahren,' Frankfurt, 1971, p. 74. The use of the term grave here is in line with the judges' characterisation of the 'schweren Tatfolgen' of the defendants. (p. 70).

- Will Chemie Grünenthal come up with a sum of money to offer as compensation to thalidomiders and their families that might approach the extent of its guilt?
- Is it certain that the company will be found guilty in the trial?
- Would it be possible to bring the trial to an end by a public call for donations to fund a foundation to which Grünenthal would pledge a substantial sum?[292]

We have already established that the answer to question one was a definite no. In contrast, we will never know the answer to question two because the trial was suspended before it was concluded. But the answer to question three is a very resounding yes. In fact, this is essentially what happened. But what was the precise mechanism for it coming about?

Here, we turn to consideration of a selection of astonishingly frank and telling documents. The first was an expert report prepared by the prosecutor's office conducting the trial sometime in spring 1969. At issue were the legal options available for suspension of the trial, which all hinged around the application of paragraph 153 III StPO of the German legal code. The prosecutors put forward four major points in support of application of the paragraph to the trial, although three of them were dismissed without much further consideration, including, interestingly enough, the possibility that all defendants would be found not guilty. The experts indicated laconically that 'this possibility does not seem apparent at this point in time'. Indeed, to the prosecutors, the only really convincing reason for applying it would be that the children affected by thalidomide would get an assured and immediate payment from Chemie Grünenthal. The experts in the prosecutor's office admitted that there were potential downsides to this, including most importantly the possibility that the firm would go into receivership before the children and their families received their payouts. This was dismissed, however, as highly unlikely, and even it were to happen, survivors would have recourse to civil suits against the Dalli group firms associated with Chemie Grünenthal.[293]

[292] Höffner to Heinemann, 28 October 1969, BArch B122/10839, Bl. 369.

[293] Expert report of the North Rhine Westphalian Justice Ministry, n.d. [ca. spring 1969], LA NRW Duisburg, Ger Rep 0139 00363, Bl. 0091-0092, quotation from Bl. 0092. In our initial evaluation of this document, we originally dated it from spring 1970 owing to a reference in it to a court decision of late November 1969 (which was apparently a typo). (See Lenhard-Schramm, 'Die Haltung,' p. 29.) The earlier dating, which we are grateful to have had corrected, still calls into question Lenhard-Schramm's contention that the prosecution was

In contrast to the minimal and unconvincing justifications for applying paragraph 153 of the legal code in order to bring the trial to an end, prosecutors put forward a raft of reasons in spring 1969 for not applying it in this case. Most of the time, they pointed out, the paragraph was used in cases involving 'insignificant crimes' or 'minor levels of guilt', which they argued was certainly not applicable here; after all, grievous bodily harm was not a minor crime. In this regard, they also pointed to the range and severity of injuries inflicted by the drug and the numbers affected, whether the damages had come in the form of polyneuritis or birth defects. Again, they suggested, the trial should continue. It was, moreover, most definitely in the 'public interest' to continue the trial for a variety of reasons, including the 'significance of the concrete deed', the 'considerable public interest in the clarification of what happened' and the issue of 'equality of treatment' before the law. Finally, the prosecutors argued 'there are good grounds to assume that most of the representatives of the co-plaintiffs would not agree to a total settlement amounting to 100 to 150 million DM and that they would deem a suspension a "scandal"'.[294]

In other words, the prosecutors were not at all convinced of the wisdom – or even the legality – of suspending the trial, certainly in spring 1969 and, as we shall demonstrate shortly, even as late as spring 1970. But this suspension happened nevertheless, with the justification that there was no 'public interest' in pursuing the trial further, i.e. in direct contradiction to the expert findings of the prosecutors. How did this come about? Here, two documents that we found in the German federal archives stand out; both are astonishing in their frankness and clearly establish the role of the federal government in linking the settlement with the end of the trial.

The first of these was a letter dated 7 April 1970 from West German President Gustav Heinemann to the Minister of Finance in the federal government, Alex Möller. The purpose of the letter was to push Möller

'längst' in favour of suspension of the trial in February 1970. What is more, a document cited by Lenhard-Schramm (pp. 605-606) from 11 March 1970 (FMJ Staatsekretär, Vermerk Betr.: Contergan, 11 March 1970, BArch B 141/59478, Bl. 152-153, quotation Bl. 152) which we will come to shortly indicates clearly continued opposition from the prosecution to this 'solution' well into spring 1970, thus undermining Lenhard-Schramm's contention that the idea of suspending the trial originated with the prosecution rather than with state or federal authorities (29). In spite of otherwise detailed recapitulations of archival sources in Lenhard-Schramm's dissertation, this very important point is not mentioned in this case.

294 Expert report of the North Rhine Westphalian Justice Ministry, n.d. [ca. spring 1969], LA NRW Duisburg, Ger Rep 0139 00363, Bl. 0093-0096.

towards making a decision about how and at what amount the federal government might contribute financially – along with Chemie Grünenthal, industry, the churches and the general public – towards the creation of a foundation to support disabled children. The plea that the federal government be involved is not surprising given Heinmann's clear interest in this matter, as established above. But what is astonishing in the document is the President's admission about what he had been up to in terms of linking a settlement to the end of the trial:

> *For months I have been involved in efforts to limit the damage from the vexatious Contergan trial by means of a financial settlement on the part of the Chemie Grünenthal firm.*[295]

He could not have been clearer about his role in helping engineer the trial's end, which would be the direct result of a financial settlement guaranteed by the firm.

But the President's letter from early April 1970 was only putting the finishing touches on a deal that was already well in place. Here, there is one more key document in this regard from about a month earlier, and it is the clearest statement by far of the exact way in which the trial was brought to a close in December 1970 as a result of the machinations of a number of actors from German politics, the legal profession and business without the participation of survivors or their representatives until at least mid-March 1970. A memorandum of 11 March 1970 (five days before the survivors and their representatives were given their first information about a proposed foundation to administer compensation), written by the State Secretary in the Federal Ministry of Justice, reported on a telephone conversation earlier that day with Baron von Münchhausen of the North Rhine Westphalian Justice Ministry. The topic at hand was whether the efforts in the direction of a 'legislative solution to the Contergan problem' would mean an end to the trial. The State Secretary was circumspect insofar as he denied that there was any way in which a financial contribution made by the firm towards a foundation would directly entail that the trial would be suspended , yet another indication that a direct connection between the two things was probably unconstitutional/illegal. But he went on to say:

[295] Letter of President Heinemann to Federal Minister of Finance (Möller), 7 April 1970 (carbon copy), Subject: 'Aid Organisation for the Disabled Child' Foundation, BArch B141/59479, Bl. 54-55.

> *...this does nothing, however, to change the fact that the firm Chemie Grünenthal could cherish the certain expectation that the criminal trial would be stopped [in the case of a financial offer], and also nothing to change the fact that in the general interest of justice the proceedings taking place in Alsdorf ... must be settled.*

In other words, there was in fact a definite connection between the settlement and the trial's end. Von Münchhausen then promised the State Secretary to have a word with the prosecutors' office in Aachen to get them to agree to suspend proceedings if 'satisfactory and reliable financial arrangements are firmly in place'. When asked if the prosecutors would be willing to do this, Münchhausen replied 'only very reluctantly' ('nur sehr ungern') (which was not surprising given the expert report from about a year earlier that we presented above), but he also stated unambiguously that the prosecutors would, *if so instructed,* certainly be relied upon to agree to the suspension of the trial and to put forward this recommendation in court.[296] In other words, the prosecutors were still not fully on board with the idea of agreeing to suspend proceedings through 11 March 1970.

Just under a week after this conversation took place, representatives of the children who were affected by thalidomide were finally invited to have their first sight of the draft legislation about a settlement involving establishment of a charitable foundation[297] which had been devised by federal government officials with direct input from Chemie Grünenthal and less direct input from the North Rhine Westphalian Justice Ministry.[298] The families would have no alternative but to agree. In the short term, a direct compensation agreement between Chemie Grünenthal and the survivors of the thalidomide disaster was signed on 10 April 1970, but it was never implemented, and was in fact, by virtue of the forthcoming legislation to create a foundation to administer funds for compensation, 'obsolete before it was even fully agreed'.[299]

[296] FMJ Staatsekretär, Vermerk Betr.: Contergan, 11 March 1970, BArch B 141/59478, Bl. 152-153, quotation Bl. 152.

[297] Memo (BMGes), Betr.: Stiftung 'Hilfswerk für das behinderte Kind', 17 March 1970, BArch B141/59479, Bl. 5-8. B141/59479, Bl. 5-8.

[298] e.g.: Wichmann to Ministerialdirector Dahlmann et. al., 13 February 1970, and attachment; 'Gesprächspartner der Arbeitsgruppe', n.d. [February 1970], both in B141/59477. Chemie Grünenthal's attorney-in-fact in these negotiations, Pick, is listed explicitly as an 'associate of Dr. Dr. Neuberger', the Justice Minister of North Rhine Westphalia and Pick's partner in his law practice.

[299] Lenhard-Schramm in 'Die Haltung', p. 630.

The day after that agreement on direct payment, on 11 April 1970, Grünenthal agreed to pay the administrative costs of the foundation in addition to its DM 100 million contribution to the foundation, and the federal government in return agreed that, when and if the families accepted this solution, it would top up the fund with an additional DM 50-100 million (although only part of this would be earmarked specifically for children damaged by thalidomide).[300] Getting everything finalised took a bit more time. When that had occurred, the trial was duly suspended on 18 December 1970.

It is worth considering the written opinion of the judges about the trial and the reasons for its suspension because it contains dimensions that are every bit as extraordinary as aspects of the trial itself. The mixed signals in the opinion constitute the first thing that is noteworthy. On the one hand, the judgment was damning: the court found the defendants culpable of 'negligence' ('fahrlässiges Verhalten') in the case of thalidomide victims who suffered nerve damage. Moreover, the court 'considers it possible that, according to that [i.e. the evidence presented], the issue of the foreseeability of malformations [of babies] would be answered in the affirmative' ('hält es für möglich, daß danach die Vorhersehbarkeit der Mißbildungen [von Babies] zu bejahen würde'). The judges also viewed the actions of the firm and its representatives as not living up to the standards which might be expected of a drug producer. On the other hand, the judges' ultimate conclusion was astonishingly: 'The court judges the guilt of each of the defendants as slight overall' ('Kammer wertet das Verschulden von jedes einzelnen Angeklagten als insgesamt gering')![301]

The same ambiguity and mixed signals held true for the lengthy list of circumstances the judges set forth as mitigating the grave misdeeds – the judges even wrote explicitly of the 'guilt' – of the defendants. For instance, they insisted that the firm's withdrawal of the drug in response to allegations that it was causing malformations in babies took place in a 'relatively short time', at least compared to the situation in Japan and other countries, but noted as well that this judgement was 'despite the unusually heavy consequences' of the defendants' misdeeds. Furthermore, the judges saw the very long period of time during which the

[300] Henning Sjöström, Robert Nilsson, *Thalidomide and the power of the drug companies*, p. 255.

[301] Medizinisch Pharmazeutische Studiengesellschaft e.V., Dokumentation III/71, 'Schriftlicher Einstellungsbeschluß der Ersten Großen Strafkammer des Landgerichts Aachen im sog. Contergan-Verfahren', Frankfurt, 1971, pp. 34-64. Quotations from (in order), pp. 34, 58 and 64.

accused were being investigated and then standing trial as a mitigating circumstance. 'The defendants have in the meantime paid off [abgetragen] a part of their guilt [sic],' the judges claimed, but at the same time they stressed that in saying this they did not overlook 'the incomparable fate of those damaged by thalidomide'. Moreover, the judges commended the defendants for having admitted their 'wrongdoing' [Fehlverhalten], while also noting that this admission was given in a 'very reserved and cautious form'. Finally, the judges counted the 'legally binding' offer of compensation to the survivors of the thalidomide catastrophe as another factor in mitigation, although here they noted that this was mainly because of likely delays in obtaining compensation through subsequent civil suits.[302]

The other bizarre aspect of the judges' written opinion involved the issue of the costs of the case. They noted that normally in the case of a suspension of a trial these costs would be covered by the state. In this particular situation, however, and quite astonishingly, Chemie Grünenthal agreed to cover all costs, including not only those incurred by the state, but also by the plaintiffs![303] Given the length of the trial, these costs must have been extraordinarily high, and it was a gesture that must have been part of the package that exchanged suspension of the trial for cash from the firm to compensate thalidomide survivors, although there seems to be no paper trail in the public archives consulted about this.

Finally, it will be useful to recount briefly some of the main findings set out in this chapter in relation to the suspension of the trial. As we have demonstrated on the basis of extensive archival evidence:

- The Wirtz family and their lawyers began to try to engineer an end to the trial by meeting with officials from the Federal Health Ministry in July 1969, offering a substantial sum to be paid to survivors through a foundation in return for the trial being suspended. From that point forward, federal government officials took a prominent role in the negotiations that culminated in just this, in spite of continued denial by the

302 *Ibid.,* pp. 70-74. Quotations from (in order) 71, 70, 71, 74.

303 *Ibid.,* p. 75. When these costs are combined with the firm's own costs for its small army of defence attorneys, its press office and so on as well as the compensation promised to the surviving children damaged by thalidomide (DM 100 million plus interest) and that promised to those affected by polyneuritis (DM 4 million), it must have exceeded the value of Chemie Grünenthal at the time.

German government which continues to the present day.[304] This was probably unconstitutional, an interpretation that is particularly likely given the insistence on the part of many of the contemporary actors in the records cited that there be no direct connection between the ending of the trial and the provision of the settlement.

- Josef Neuberger, the former defence attorney for Hermann Wirtz who became Justice Minister of North Rhine Westphalia in December 1966, also played a prominent role in these negotiations through his state secretary, Baron von Münchhausen, who liaised closely with officials from the federal government and representatives of Chemie Grünenthal in engineering a settlement in return for suspension of the trial. During the run-up to and during the course of the trial, Neuberger was also involved in an ongoing basis through his associates in his law practice, which continued to provide defence attorney services to the most prominent Grünenthal defendants and to serve as consultants for the firm in negotiations to create a charitable foundation to dispense compensation funds. This represented at best extreme conflict of interest, and was probably also unconstitutional.
- The prosecution conducting the trial was actively opposed to its suspension through at least spring 1969 and was extremely reluctant to go down this path as late as spring 1970.
- The deal to suspend the trial in return for compensation offered by the firm and administered through a charitable foundation was worked out by representatives of Chemie Grünenthal in conjunction with officials from the state government of North Rhine Westphalia and the German federal government. Representatives of the families of survivors were intentionally excluded from these negotiations until they had effectively been concluded in March 1970.

After the details were worked out in the coming months, the trial was duly suspended on 18 December 1970 and a law enabling the establishment of the foundation was passed just a day short of a year later. All in all, it is clear that the results of this enormous fight for

304 Letter from Elke Ferner Parliamentarische Staatssekretärin im BMFSFJ to Mr. Neil Parish MP dated Berlin, 8 April 2014.

justice in Germany against the firm that was primarily responsible for producing and marketing thalidomide – a company that moreover continued doing so in the face of mounting evidence of the harm it was doing, denying falsely all the time that it was not in possession of such evidence – were unacceptable to say the least. The settlement was offered reluctantly and on the basis of a clear strategy for limiting liability. Even more importantly, for those directly affected it was utterly inadequate. It was a deal engineered by the German federal government involving interference in a criminal trial, which privileged the interests of a few powerful industrialists over those of a very large number of less advantaged and well-connected individuals who had been harmed irreparably by the product of the firm at the centre of all of this, Chemie Grünenthal. This was, though, only the first round in the fight for justice for thalidomiders and their families. The next round was not long in coming, although the struggle for adequate compensation and for clear recognition of responsibility and guilt on the part of those responsible for the thalidomide disaster continues to the present.

Chapter Seven

Trying for Justice (2)

'Ich bin ein Produkt von Grünenthal.'

AS NIGHT WAS FALLING ON SUNDAY, 30 September 2007, a motley group of people began to gather on Zweifaller Strasse in the pretty, old Rhineland town of Stolberg. Some were in wheelchairs; some had short and deformed arms and hands; others had ears missing and paralysed faces. They gathered outside the gate of the old Chemie Grünenthal factory for a vigil that was to last until the following Monday morning, 1 October 2007. Many wore T-shirts with the slogan 'Ich bin ein Produkt von Grünenthal' ('I am a product of Grünenthal') on the front; on the back was a call for a boycott of a range of products manufactured by other companies owned by the Wirtz family, the proprietors of Chemie Grünenthal, including the perfume brands Tabac, Nonchalance, Tosca and 4711. The timing was significant: 1 October 2007 marked the 50th anniversary of the official sales launch of Contergan and thus also of the beginning of the catastrophe. The main organiser of the event, Andreas Meyer, was a four-limb damaged thalidomider who had been battling for many years to try to secure a better deal for all the German Contergan survivors.

Monika Eisenberg-Geginat has described how it felt to take part in this as well as earlier and later vigils:

> *When I was 16 years old I went to Stolberg for the first time. I looked at the front gate of the Grünenthal factory. I wanted to rattle on that gate and make them face what they had done to me, my body, my family, my friends. How could it be that Grünenthal could go on producing drugs and the Wirtz family*

owners had a trouble-free life? Why was there no justice for us? Why was there no justice for us and our families? Of course I didn't rattle on that gate that day – I was only 16 and I was angry and anxious and very young.

Figure 11: Black Balloons at Stolberg, 1st October 1987.

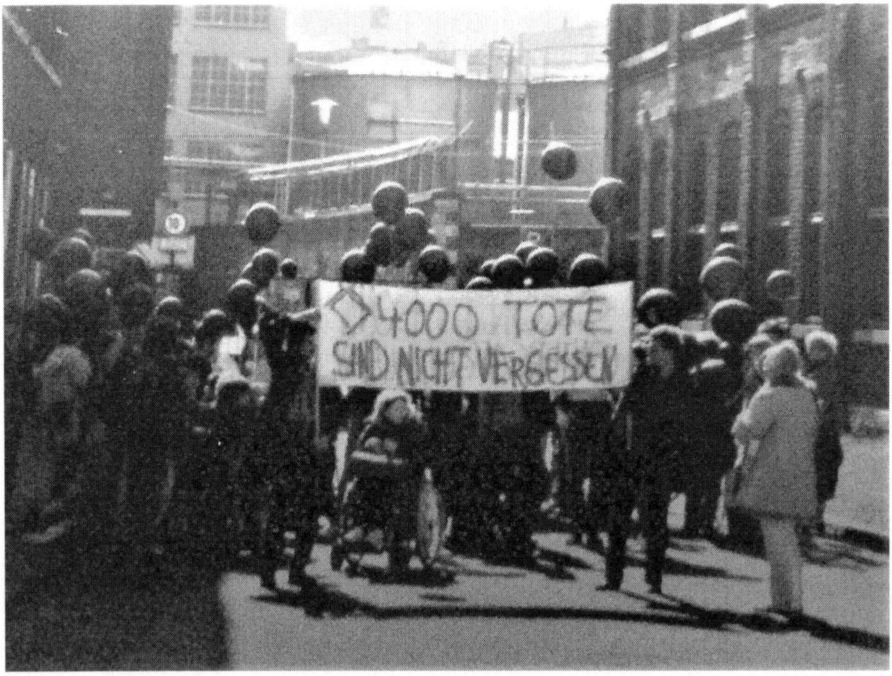

© M Eisenberg-Geginat

After some years many Contergan survivors went to Stolberg. That was the night of September 30th to October 1st 1987, the 30th anniversary of launching the drug on the market. Andreas Meyer, a survivor from Cologne, called on the Contergan survivors to go to Stolberg for a silent vigil in remembrance of the 5000 babies who didn't survive the first year. We spent a very cold night there but the atmosphere was dignified. For the first time we formed the word Contergan with red grave candles and kept the lights on the whole night. I thought, it will brighten the remembrance of each dead victim. I wished them to be little angels and have a fantastic time wherever they were. But we kept the fire on also for us, for our life. The whole night there was not a single reaction from the company and the building was dark apart of a row of lights on the first floor. The next day we made a demonstration walk from the company to the marketplace and we made speeches. The Wirtz family lives in a wonderful house near the market. Everybody had a black balloon in his hand or on the wheelchair. After our event we let the balloons fly as a symbol for so many souls who were not with us and will never be. This was the first vigil.

We returned for the next vigil in 1997. We had the red grave candles and formed the word Contergan like before. That was again on the night of September 30th to October 1st. We had white flowers with us, and this time we laid a wreath in front of the gate. We laid the flowers in a criss-cross pattern on the street. We kept the candles burning the whole night. Survivors came with their families, children and friends. The atmosphere was different to the first one – but we showed we are still here. It was very sombre. Next day, for Grünenthal another working day started, but some of us were still there talking and packing stuff, fixing up the wreath and rearranging the flower pattern on the street. The first truck came out of the company gate but we moved the wreath so that the truck could pass. The driver was not able to drive over the flowers. I saw tears running over his face. I was very sorry for him. It hit the wrong person. No word from Grünenthal.

We returned for the next vigil in 2007, on the 50th anniversary of Contergan coming on the market. In the meantime, Grünenthal had pulled down some of the houses in that street in front of the gate. The place was more open. We hired a big tent with some chairs, so everybody could go into the warmth. We laid a wreath again and the flowers. But we also put up posters with pictures of Sebastian Wirtz who was now the manager of the company. We wrote on the posters our needs and our anger about so many lies and fraud. After the first vigil I was not anxious anymore. Now it is all about revenge. All the years, lies, fraud, blatant injustice. Grünenthal started to make everything very nice for themselves with a new factory in Eilendorf and new office buildings. We all had T-shirts on, printed: 'I am a product of Grünenthal'.

We returned to another vigil in 2009. Grünenthal offered us a tent and there were people with hot drinks and soup to stay through the night. A tent for our pains and our suffering and, and, and... no words. We held speeches and put flags from all countries with Thalidomide survivors on the gate. We kept the candles burning but there is also a fire burning inside me – the fire let me be thirsty for justice and dignity ... but also I want revenge. So many times I have been back to Stolberg. The Wirtz family pulled down the early headquarters of Grünenthal in the street where the house of the family is... but they cannot pull down the truth and our memories. Our destinies and their guilt will stick to them. They are guilty and killed children and destroyed families. Guilty of causing my pains.

Wenn die Wahrheit zu schwach ist, sich zu verteidigen, dann muss sie zum Angriff übergehen. (When truth is too weak to defend itself, it must go on the attack.) – Bertholt Brecht.[305]

Initial quests for compensation

To be fair, truth actually went on the offensive very quickly after the withdrawal of thalidomide from most markets in 1961, and, to a greater or lesser degree, truth has been on the attack ever since. But as the anger and frustration so palpable in Monika Eisenberg-Geginat's testimony make clear, the struggle for some sort of justice has been both protracted and elusive. And the initial attempts to gain compensation and admission of responsibility proved agonizingly difficult, not least because the results eventually achieved were as inadequate and unsatisfactory as they were grudgingly granted.

In the first round, which lasted from 1961 until the early 1970s, compensation agreements were reached in four of the key countries involved in the tragedy: Sweden (where the first settlement was reached), Germany, the UK and Japan. But this happened only after protracted legal wrangling, during which time survivors and their families had to fend for themselves as the companies involved sought to protect their assets by refusing admission of liability, mainly in the first instance by disputing the causal link between the drug and its effects on

[305] Testimony of Monika Eisenberg-Geginat, Contergan survivor, Cologne, 21 February 2014.

disabled children. And remember that many survivors died during this time.

Figure 12: Monika Eisenberg-Geginat, Educational Psychologist, aged 20.

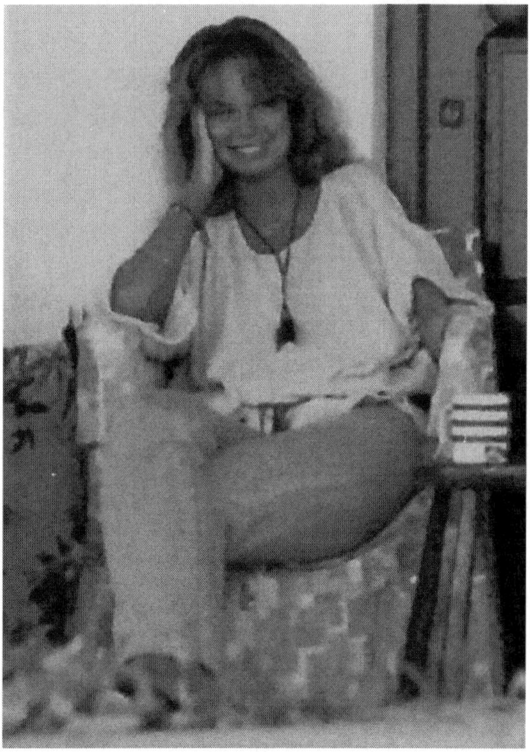

© M. Eisenberg-Geginat

The first trial of one of the companies associated with the thalidomide disaster involved a civil lawsuit filed in Sweden, where the Swedish Medical Board had cleared the drug for sale by the Astra pharmaceutical company. Astra had concluded a licensing agreement with Grünenthal in March 1957 that gave the Swedish firm sole rights for sales of thalidomide in Scandinavia.[306] Even here in the earliest attempt at justice, delay was the order of the day; the trial did not begin until December 1965, and it took nearly four years before a settlement was finally concluded in October 1969. This resulted in a fund of 68 million Swedish kronor (at the time to be divided among 100 children who had suffered thalidomide damage). A few Danish victims were

[306] Henning Sjöström, Robert Nilsson, *Thalidomide and the power of the drug companies,* p. 38.

added to this settlement, and a separate but parallel agreement was made for the few thalidomide survivors identified in Norway. At 1969 currency exchange rates, the total funds available to the victims thus corresponded to about £5.5 million.[307] At approximately £55,000 per person on average, this was easily the most generous of the initial settlements in major Western countries, although even the Swedish amount proved woefully inadequate over the long term.

Germany, on the other hand, differed from Sweden not only in featuring a far less generous initial settlement, but also by virtue of the fact that there were criminal as well as civil legal proceedings there. Germany was also the only country where the government co-financed the initial compensation scheme for thalidomide victims, a scheme which was eventually launched in the early 1970s. The quest for some sort of compensation started already, however, in the immediate aftermath of the drug's withdrawal from sale in November 1961, with many individual claims lodged in the form of civil lawsuits. But these were overtaken in the latter part of the decade by the trial of company staff for criminal charges ranging from manslaughter to causing bodily injury to adult and child victims. As we have seen in Chapter 6, Chemie Grünenthal eventually put an offer of 100 million deutschmarks (just under £10 million at 1969 exchange rates[308]) on the table for the German survivors of thalidomide, which was larger in absolute terms than the Swedish settlement but, given the much greater number of survivors in Germany, amounted to far less per person. Indeed, it amount to less than DM 40,000 (£4,064) per person on average. To add insult to injury, the company made the offer subject to a guarantee that the firm would not ever be faced with any additional legal or financial liabilities in conjunction with the catastrophe. It insisted that the criminal trial of its executives stopped as well. Chapter 6 also describes the growing involvement of the German federal government in the whole business of arranging a settlement package, which led to an agreement being brokered to end the trial. The federal government also topped up Grünenthal's offer with an additional contribution of DM 110 million and was instrumental in the establishment of a foundation to administer the compensation scheme, the framework of which was

[307] Based on exchange rates between British pound sterling and Swedish krona in 1969 at: *http://fx.sauder.ubc.ca/etc/GBPpages.pdf* <viewed 25 March 2015>.
[308] Based on exchange rates between British pound sterling and Deutschmark in 1969 at: *http://fx.sauder.ubc.ca/etc/GBPpages.pdf* <viewed 25 March 2015>.

established through legislation enacted on 17 December 1971, a day short of the first anniversary of the suspension of the trial. The government contribution, however, was not earmarked exclusively for the victims of thalidomide. Instead, only DM 50 million of the DM 110 million it put forward went to them, with remaining funds made available to members of other disability groups.[309] The 'fudge' here was reflected in the very name of the foundation finally set up in 1972: the Stiftung Hilfswerk für behinderte Kinder (Foundation 'Aid Organisation for Disabled Children'), which operated as a quasi-governmental agency under the auspices of the Pensions Ministry. Indeed, it was not until October 2005 that the connection to thalidomide was made explicit when the foundation was renamed the Conterganstiftung für behinderte Menschen (the Contergan Foundation for Disabled People), finally linking the foundation's real purpose through inclusion of Chemie Grünenthal's trade name for thalidomide.[310]

A key point here is how woefully inadequate the foundation as it existed from 1972 to the early 21st century was in terms of compensation for victims. Here is the context: there were about 2,600 registered thalidomide claimants in Germany (and eventually 2,901 from Germany and five other countries who were registered with the foundation through 2011[311]). Furthermore, as mentioned already, at the outset only DM 160 million of the foundation's total capital of DM 220 million was available to thalidomiders. The total funding from the combination of the company's contribution (indicated above on a per capita basis) and from the government therefore amounted to DM 61,538 (£7,727) per German survivor of the drug on average, and to DM 55,153 (£6,929)[312] on average if all of those registered by the early 21st century with the German foundation are taken into account. Depending on which of these two figures we use, this amounted to just 12.6%-14% of the average Swedish settlement per survivor. To put it in

309 Summary details are available at: *http://www.fr-online.de/panorama/hintergrund-der-contergan-skandal,1472782,2704116.html* <viewed 10 February 2016>. The two classes of beneficiaries are indicated in the text of the law as amended through 2002: Gesetz über die Errichtung einer Stiftung 'Hilfswerk für behinderte Kinder' StHG) vom 17. Dezember 1971 Stand: 9. Änderungsgesetz vom 21.6.2002.

310 Gesetz über die Stiftung für Behinderte Menschen (Contergan Stiftungsgesetz ContStifG) vom 13 Okt 2005.

311 Based on figures collated by the Thalidomide Trust 2001-2013 from a variety of sources, including reports from the Conterganstiftung.

312 Based on exchange rates between British pound sterling and the Deutschmark in 1972 at: *http://fx.sauder.ubc.ca/etc/GBPpages.pdf* <viewed 25 March 2015>.

another perspective, under either of these two compensation schemes, but by far worse in the German one, often severely disable people had access to a more or less insufficient total sum of money that needed to be drawn upon over the course of their entire lives. As a result, annual payouts to thalidomide survivors in Germany were very low indeed, and even so the fund ran out of money in 1997. The German federal government 'solved' the problem of erosion of capital by funding the foundation from its annual budget beginning that same year. Even so, as late as 2007, the maximum payout from the German fund for individual Contergan survivors was only €545 per month for even the most severely damaged.[313] To put this sum in perspective, this was only about 20% of the amount received per month during that year by a survivor with four-limb damage who was registered with the UK Thalidomide Trust.

But we get ahead of ourselves a bit. After all, the initial offer of compensation in the UK was none too generous either. To begin with, Distillers put an offer on the table of £3,250,000 that would be divided up among the full group of about 430 children, which worked out at an average of just over £7,500 each.[314] It was a take-it-or-leave it offer that, based on the current exchange rates, was very close to the average amount per survivor awarded in the eventual German settlement arrived at between 1970 and 1972 when the federal government stepped in to top up the original Chemie Grünenthal offer.[315] There was, though, a major difference between the 'final' Distillers' offer and the funding that went into the German foundation. In Britain, a strong and effective public relations and media campaign forced an increase of more than five times in the amount that Distillers actually paid survivors compared to its initial offer, amounting to a total of £20 million in 1973. This meant that the funding available for British victims was about six times as much per survivor as was available per affected child under the German settlement. By this point, the British settlement amounted to about 85% of the Swedish one (£46,512 vs.

[313] Key word 'Stiftung' linked to article by Gregor Taxacher, 'Erfolgsstory mit katastrophalem Makel', *Westdeutsche Rundfunk* (23 November 2006). Available at: *http://www.wdr.de/themen/gesundheit/pharmazie/contergan/gruenenthal.jhtml#sw05* <viewed 24 March 2009>.

[314] *The Sunday Times* Insight Team, *Suffer The Children: The Story of Thalidomide,* pp. 161-164.

[315] The average amount per survivor in Germany translated into £7,727 when the Foundation was established in 1972, while the Distillers offer in 1971 had been increased slightly from the company's initial one to £8,140. We have calculated the German amount based on exchange rates in 1972 at: *http://fx.sauder.ubc.ca/etc/GBPpages.pdf* <viewed 25 March 2015>.

£54,768 on average[316]), but both were vastly better than the fund available to German victims. The inescapable conclusion of the eventual outcome of the British negotiations is that Distillers originally believed they could get away with the same derisory level of settlements as Grünenthal had until the media storm led by *The Sunday Times,* under its then editor, Harold Evans, made this impossible.[317]

In any event, like the German one, the British settlement agreed in 1973 also resulted in the establishment of a foundation, although there were major differences in organisation and in procedures. For instance, unlike the German settlement, the British one provided for a lump-sum payment according to the relative degree of disability for each child, and also provided £5,000 for each set of parents. The balance of £14 million was used to create a fund to be administered by the Thalidomide Trust, on the basis that it was, for practical purposes, impossible to know in advance just what the needs of the children were going to be in future years.

In Japan, the last of the countries we look at here, a foundation was established in 1974 by agreement between the manufacturer of the drug, Dainippon, and the Japanese government. The Ishizue foundation has since provided annual funding to the 309 thalidomide survivors who have been identified. The parents were awarded sums equating to £12,500 each, while between £104,000 and £154,000 was made available to each child depending on the severity of injuries. The total value of this settlement in 1974 was approximately £42 million.[318] All in all, then, by these arduous and protracted means, settlements eventually reached in Sweden, Germany, the UK and Japan all provided payments to the children whose disabilities were recognised as having been caused by thalidomide. But, significantly, it took an average of ten years to get to this stage, during which time about 75% of the children born alive with thalidomide damage passed away; these children and their families never benefitted from the eventual settlement. Moreover, for all of the families affected, the whole process involved an apparently never-ending legal battle that often broke families and relationships.

[316] Based on exchange rates between British pound sterling and Swedish krona in 1969 for the Swedish settlement and in 1973 for the British one at: *http://fx.sauder.ubc.ca/etc/GBPpages.pdf* <viewed 25 March 2015>.

[317] *The Sunday Times* Insight Team, *Suffer The Children: The Story of Thalidomide,* pp. 182-203.

[318] Report by Professor Tsugumichi Sato, Ishizue Foundation director, to Thalidomide Trust, September 2009. The report gives compensation figures in US dollars, and these have been converted using the 1974 exchange rate for US$: £1 = $2.40.

Michael Carr-Jones, one of the founders of the British campaign group (which eventually became the Thalidomide Society), has written about this aspect of the experience, and his views are worth quoting at some length:

> *I personally brought the first writ to Distillers through my Solicitors Kimber Bull. We were distraught and I helped form an association of parents, I was Chairman and we had, as a figurehead, the wife of Lord Mayor of London, Mary Hoare (Lady Hoare).*
>
> *I visited Germany for the first time and there were hundreds of children born like Graham. I had always an inbuilt dislike of all things German, a relic of the war, I suppose, but I was both delighted and amazed to find them better friends than I could imagine. I remember visiting and finding many things that would be useful in UK for our children and was astonished at the reprimand I received from Lady Hoare telling me to be 'more British' this was one of many occasions when I was aware that her and my basic goal was so different. She became our president by default but she had a passionate dislike of the litigation we were planning it was a taboo subject. Not only litigation but commercialism, I recall one Christmas when we were offered the support of several stars (including) Tommy Steele and Dora Bryan. Peter Carter and I went to see Lady Hoare at the Mansion House where she was at a dinner full of excitement about this so generous offer and she turned it down flat as too commercial!*
>
> *It was amazing to us how the press treated us, I lobbied several MPs and was disgusted with the offhand treatment I was given. I wrote to Gerald Nabarro (Very high profile and wealthy MP), I asked him to lobby for special allowances for our children. He said he was fed up with snivelling parents always trying to get money. I waited for hours to see Jeremy Thorpe (Liberal Party leader) and he finally sent me a message that he was too busy to see me. A big contrast with Mary Wilson (wife of Harold Wilson, Prime Minister) who offered her help as long as it did not tread on the toes of Lady Hoare.*

I recall that the day we went public in the press asking for funds to help parents in their predicament we had hardly any response, but an Alsatian dog caught his paw on a railway track and the owners received over £800 in unsolicited donations.

Many Mothers unable to cope committed suicide and the famous Mother in Bruges Belgium murdered her child. The Daily Mail *phoned me at 2.30 in the morning of the story and asked what I thought. They misquoted me when I said 'they are not freaks you know' and they left out the word 'not'. I had a meeting with the parents next day and you can imagine the stick I got for that. The newspapers were reluctant to print our stories when we placed them as so many of the papers relied on Distillers for advertising revenue. It seemed like a huge uphill struggle. I was closely involved with the parents, the legal proceedings and the press and TV and giving talks right left and centre, I lived and breathed this for nearly 13 years and had so much help from unexpected quarters and surprisingly little from where you would expect. I had so much support from my wife Norma and my brother Gordon, otherwise I would not have been able to do all I did.*

Enoch Powell, Health Minister in the Conservative Government, and I met when we had a meeting at the Ministry of Health during the time we were trying to get more help for the Thalidomide Children. I never met a more cold person. We were at this meeting and one of the parents of a victim of Distaval asked if it would be possible to use Powell's influence to get a prescription for an insect repellent for her armless daughter who was being plagued by insects in the garden. The family in question were not well enough off to buy these things and Enoch Powell in my presence along with others just swept her on one side and said 'that is not open to discussion here'. We were all open mouthed at the arrogance of the man.

At first Gerald Gardiner a very eminent QC agreed to act for us, unfortunately he was then made Lord Chief Justice which was great for him but he had to turn us over to a colleague Desmond Ackner. From then on it all went downhill. He had an offer from Distillers to settle. We called a meeting of the litigants and he

> *asked me to persuade them to accept the offer telling me and them that this offer was the best we could hope for and if we did not accept that would be that, it was a terrible time and we were bullied into accepting. I was not surprised to see Desmond Ackner become a Lord soon after, bearing out my suspicion that there was a lot going on behind the scenes that we were not aware of. I was away in Wales for a long week end when I had a phone call saying that Kimber Bull had been told that my personal claim had to be settled by noon Friday or it would be dismissed. It was Thursday when I got the message and having been in litigation for nearly 12 years to have that many hours to rush things through was not gentle.*[319]

If, though, the 25% of thalidomide children born alive in these four countries who lived long enough for the hard-won settlements to be reached got some benefit – however inadequate – from the funds, children in many other countries where thalidomide had been distributed (mainly under licence) fared far less well. In Italy, for instance, the drug was widely used, resulting in around 350 survivors who have been identified there. But all six Italian companies known to have sold thalidomide went out of business before they could be forced to pay compensation. As a result, none of the 350 Italian survivors received settlement at all until the government finally stepped in to provide some benefits starting in 2008. In Spain, on the other hand, where the drug had been sold directly by Grünenthal and two other companies, government authorities denied flatly that the drug had ever been used there until they had a change of heart in 2007,[320] this in spite of the fact that the German foundation had long recognised three Spanish survivors as eligible for benefits under its scheme. The new Spanish government scheme had admitted 23 more Spanish thalidomide survivors following a law passed in 2010 which provided funding of, on average, less than €70,000 each. And this figure covered no more than a handful of the possible Spanish cases: local estimates conclude that there could have been as many as 1,000 survivors in all.[321]

[319] Michael Carr-Jones, private correspondence with Martin Johnson, 24 January 2012; 7 February 2012.

[320] 'Spain's Forgotten Thalidomiders', *BBC News* report 1 November 2007, viewed on 22 December 2015 at: *http://news.bbc.co.uk/1/hi/programmes/crossing_continents/7067839.stm*

[321] DLA Piper survey; report for the Conterganstiftung January 2012 pp. 93-94 (Italy); 197-200 (Spain).

In a variety of countries in Latin America, survivors found no recourse to compensation at all. For example, a DLA Piper survey of 2010-2012 commissioned by the German Conterganstiftung came to this conclusion in its report on the situation in Mexico:

> *Following an extensive examination of the publicly accessible sources, in particular public health statistics and sources of the Mexican government, it is impossible to identify publicly documented cases of thalidomide impairment in Mexico. Relevant data do not exist and were not compiled at any time ... However, our research revealed that there seem to have been some cases of thalidomide victims in Mexico. Regarding the verification of this information, we predominantly had to rely on personal information from employees of the health authorities, newspaper articles as well as interviews with two Mexican thalidomide victims. We could gain information from a newspaper article from 1963 that the Mexican government claimed that the drug Contergan was not sold officially in Mexico... Regardless of this, it is known that thalidomide was sold in Mexico under the name Thalargan.*[322]

The Mexican situation is similar to that of many other countries in the region, with Brazil being the only exception in providing compensation to victims, although here, too, the wait has been long. Even the admission that there were problems with the drug took longer to be recognised than elsewhere. After all, in Brazil, the drug was not even taken off the market until 1965. Moreover, even after that it has notoriously continued to be used to treat ENL, a complication of leprosy. The legal battle against the manufacturer and the Brazilian government was also long delayed; it did not begin even until 1976. Proceedings then concluded in the first instance with an Act of Parliament in 1982 that created a system of life-long pension payments funded by the government and administered by the Brazilian National Security Institute. In 2012, payments went on a regular basis to around 600 thalidomide survivors, the youngest of whom was born in 2010.[323]

The situation in Canada and Australia was different again. There, survivors reached settlements on an individual basis, settlements which varied considerably according to the competence and determination of

[322] *Ibid.*, p. 123.
[323] *Ibid.*, pp. 30-33.

the lawyers who handled each case. It was not until the beginning of the 21st century, with the arrival of the Internet, that things began to change towards a more comprehensive settlement in these countries and elsewhere. By then, survivors all over Europe and in the wider world had started comparing and considering their situations. All became painfully aware that they had been sold short, let down. And many of them were determined to do something about it. The renewed campaign for justice started in the UK, with the successor to Distillers (Guinness, and then Diageo), the government and politicians the first focus of attack. Simultaneously, though, the campaign in Germany increased its level of activism, building on the vigils in Stolberg described at the start of the chapter, which had started in 1987 and continued at ten-year intervals thereafter to mark the anniversary of the start of sales of thalidomide in Germany. The British campaign was the first to bear fruit in a big way, but there was some progress in Germany, too. Both campaigns had as their ultimate target Chemie Grünenthal, which, to the surprise of many in the UK in particular, turned out to remain a wealthy and thriving business, still in the hands of its family shareholders. Let's look first at the unfolding of the new campaign in Britain before looking at the progress of the German campaign and the ways the effects of both have spread to other countries.

UK campaigns

Campaigning for justice for British thalidomiders carried on at a much lower level in the aftermath of the original 1973 settlement with Distillers, and there were, as a result, few major new developments in the two decades that followed. This, though, started to change in the early 1990s. Once again, a successful media campaign worked to force a top-up of the funds available to thalidomide victims, and the proximate cause of the new media activity was a report by actuaries advising the Thalidomide Trust which showed the funds then held would be exhausted by 2006. This news prompted beneficiary campaigners, particularly Freddie Astbury and Gary Skyner, to start a media campaign for additional funding from Guinness, the company that took over Distillers in 1986. Serendipitously, but luckily, their campaign coincided with news emerging in the first years of the 1990s of a scandal surrounding the 1986 takeover, which culminated in

Guinness directors put on trial for fraud in 1993.[324] As a result of renewed pressure from thalidomide campaigners in the wake of this scandal,[325] Guinness agreed in 1995 to provide a total of £37.5 million in additional funding through 2009 in 15 instalments of £2.5 million each. This was better than before, of course. But on the other hand, all it did was enable the Thalidomide Trust to maintain payments to survivors at existing levels, without even allowing for increases for inflation.

And so the campaign continued. The trust began collecting medical evidence to show the level of health deterioration over time among its beneficiaries, and in 1999 this was presented to Diageo plc (the company which resulted from the merger between Guinness and Grand Metropolitan). Further media campaigning, again led by Freddie Astbury and Gary Skyner, took place, and included a public call for a boycott of Diageo brands fronted by a group of prominent sportsmen.[326] Again, the pressure paid off: negotiations between the Thalidomide Trust and Diageo plc resulted in 2000 in an extension of the £2.5 million funding per year beyond 2009 through to 2022, in other words an additional commitment of £32.5 million. Moreover, this time the company agreed to index payments so that they would rise in line with inflation. So it was not until 2000, nearly 40 years after the initial withdrawal of the drug, that the beneficiaries of the Thalidomide Trust could feel any confidence that their funding was on a secure basis. Even at the start of the new millennium, though, it was clear the financial support they received still was not commensurate in any way with the actual amounts they needed to cope with their disabilities. And this was before anyone started considering the likely health deterioration to be expected among a group of thalidomiders after the age of 40.

One of the problems in this regard was that many of the beneficiaries of the Thalidomide Trust did not receive their full benefits because, surprisingly enough, the Thalidomide Trust was required to deduct tax from payments if thalidomiders took them in the form of income for beneficiaries. The Inland Revenue came to this unexpected ruling in 1973, after the agreements to establish the Trust had been finalised. The consequence was that these payments were taxed at the Combined Trusts taxation rate, which, during the time after 1974, was

324 'Last Guinness scandal trial begins', *The Independent,* 12 January 1993.
325 'Thalidomide Pressure Grows', *The Independent,* 3 March 1994.
326 'Don't Buy Them', *Daily Express,* 29 February 2000.

as high as 48%, but even in 2000 amounted to 34%. The tax could be avoided only for that portion of the funding that beneficiaries took for 'disability-related' purposes, such as vehicles, adaptations to the home or workplace or special housing. If the beneficiaries needed the money to live on, however, they had to pay income tax on it at what was, in effect, the highest combined tax rate applicable to any UK resident during those years. Therefore, the most disabled people with the least support from family or spouses, and who had the greatest need for money for food and heating, paid the highest amount of tax.

In an early attempt to mitigate this problem, the government had paid in a sum of £5 million when the Trust began it operations. Following the agreement with Guinness in 1995, John Major's government paid a further £7 million into the Trust. However, while this funding supported the overall funding level available for distribution by the Trust, it also failed to assist the beneficiaries liable to paying the high rate of income tax. In 2000, Gary Skyner suggested to the trustees that a similar offset payment should be sought from the government in conjunction with the Diageo settlement that was reached that year, for which he had campaigned very vigorously. They then approached Major, by now the former Prime Minister but still serving in parliament as MP for Huntingdonshire, the area where the Trust's office was located. Representatives of the Trust asked him to lobby for this on their behalf. He in turn wrote in February 2001 to Gordon Brown, then Chancellor of the Exchequer, requesting a further offset payment from the Labour government like the one that had been awarded under Major's government. Under the circumstances, a positive response was expected. Instead, it took eighteen months and several follow-up letters and enquiries to get a reply from Gordon Brown. When the reply finally came, it was extremely disappointing: Brown refused the request.[327]

His refusal was picked up by the *Daily Mirror,* and a feature article appeared on 26 September 2002, with the front page opening to the story carrying the headline, 'Cruel Tax'.[328] The feature story pointed out that even allowing for previous offset payments, the British government had gained a net profit of about £3 million on tax deducted

327 Letter 3 July 2002 from Gordon Brown to Rt. Hon. John Major, copied to Jonathan Djanogly MP. (Copy held by Martin Johnson.)

328 *Daily Mirror,* 26 September 2002; Articles 'Cruel Tax', 'Voice of the Daily Mirror: Stop taxing thalidomide victims now', 'We're not living the High life… and this is treating us all like deviants', authors Gary Jones and Ian Miller.

by the Thalidomide Trust from payments to beneficiaries. What is more, the paper reported, if tax deductions continued as before, the government's net profit would increase by a further £20 million during the period of the new Diageo agreement. Unsurprisingly, there was widespread outrage at the idea of the government generating revenue from the thalidomide tragedy.

At about the same time, the nature of the campaign changed dramatically because of the appearance on the scene by the end of 2002 of a new group of beneficiary campaigners led by Nick Dobrik.[329] A Cambridge University economics graduate and a successful businessman, Nick had never paid close attention to the Trust before; he was busy taking care of his business affairs, and the payments he received from it formed only a very minor part of his financial portfolio. But the unfolding of the 'Cruel Tax' story caught his attention because it highlighted the difficulties being experienced by other thalidomiders in the UK. The fact that the Labour government was apparently unwilling to help alleviate these difficulties in part by changing tax regulations was particularly galling to him as an active Labour Party member. He resolved to do something about it by working with other thalidomiders in close cooperation with the trustees and staff of the trust. He thus facilitated the creation of the first integrated thalidomide campaign in the UK led from the front by the thalidomiders themselves. The new group, closely supported by Trust staff, began an intensive lobby of members of Parliament, while the trustees used their connections to get expert legal advice. By the end of 2003, the new tactics paid off: the Treasury staff agreed that it would follow the legal advice received by the trustees and change the law. The legislation was finally enacted in August 2004.[330] From that point, the Thalidomide Trust stopped having to deduct tax from any of their payments to beneficiaries. The UK was brought into line with most other countries where thalidomiders received payments from settlement schemes without having to pay tax.

The new campaigners' victory in getting the government to change its tax policy put more money in the pockets of those beneficiaries of the Trust who were most in need. But it did not address the longstanding and still unresolved issue of the inadequacy of funds

[329] Andrew Jack, 'Thalidomide: It's Not Over Yet', *Financial Times Magazine* (22/23 September 2007).

[330] UK Government Statutory Instrument 2004 No. 1819; The Thalidomide Children's Trust (Application of Section 329AA of the Income and Corporation Taxes Act 1988) Order 2004.

available to the Trust. After all, the 2000 agreement between the Trust and Diageo extended the length of time during which funding would be forthcoming and provided for annual uplifts in funding in line with inflation, but it offered no scope for increases in benefits, which, because of the deterioration in health in aging thalidomiders, were required. So, the UK thalidomide campaigners turned their energies towards gaining an enhanced overall level of funding, aiming to get it doubled in real terms from 2004 levels. Their efforts quickly bore fruit: in 2005, Diageo plc agreed a package valued then at £168 million, which would enable the Trust to double the real value of its payments over a 17-year period to 2022. An additional series of payments from Diageo is now scheduled to run until 2037.

The movement goes international by targeting national governments

The new and enhanced payment scheme negotiated with Diageo was implemented in 2006, at a time when Thalidomide Trust staff members were in the process of actively building links with other thalidomide organisations in Europe in order to identify medical and healthcare expertise to support the rapid physical deterioration of many beneficiaries. This was paralleled by an internationalisation of campaigning as, in 2006-2007, UK campaigners started to share their experiences with those of other thalidomide groups, and especially in Germany and Sweden. Initial meetings led to a decision by thalidomide representatives from all over Europe and as far away as Canada to join forces. Accordingly, on 30 January 2008, at a meeting in the Churchill Hotel in London's West End convened under the guidance of veteran campaigner Jonathan Stone, delegates agreed to start campaigning together under the name 'International Contergan Thalidomide Alliance', or ICTA. This was a movement rather than an organisation, with activists united by their shared ultimate objective of achieving justice, and with Chemie Grünenthal as their main target. We will return shortly to the thus far futile attempts to achieve that goal of holding Chemie Grünenthal to account. The focus here at the moment is on the successful campaigns of national groups affiliated with ICTA in holding governments to account, campaigns fought of necessity at the national level, but successful in no small part because the national campaigners were talking to one another across borders. In this case, the first successful breakthrough came in Germany, although by way of London and inspired by the vigils in Stolberg.

In the Bundestag

The first main ICTA event was a demonstration outside the German Embassy in London on 3 April 2008, marking the public commencement of the new international campaign.[331] One of the main features of the day was the acknowledgement of the thousands of thalidomide children who had died, mostly never receiving any financial compensation. A cloud of black balloons, first seen just over twenty years earlier over Stolberg at the first thalidomide vigil in 1987, was released over London that day in their memory.

Through these and other initiatives, campaigners were making the point that the German government needed to do more for the survivors of the thalidomide disaster. The federal government soon recognised the merits of the case, announcing that from 1 July 2008 all payments from the German Foundation would double, which made the maximum monthly benefit payment €1,090 per month for the most severely damaged. It was a lot better than it had been since the founding of the German Foundation in 1972, but it was still only about 40% of the amount received by British thalidomiders. In addition, the German government convened a parliamentary committee meeting in Berlin on 28 May 2008, in part to discuss the impact of a €50 million donation to the German Foundation pledged that month by Grünenthal, a donation prompted in no small part by pressure exerted by the thalidomiders' campaign for justice in Germany and elsewhere that we will return to later in the chapter. One speaker at the meeting remarked succinctly, summarising the general view among campaigners and many others that this was again woefully inadequate: 'It doesn't even cover the dental expenses of 2,800 German thalidomiders.' Moving on to discussions of other matters having an impact on, and of concern to, the survivor community, the committee explored the health and other problems currently being experienced by many thalidomiders, and also heard from medical experts and a senior official of the UK Thalidomide Trust, Alan Summerside. Many of the questions raised by the committee revolved around the health conditions of the thalidomide survivors, and

331 *http://www.theguardian.com/society/2008/apr/04/health.medicalresearch* <viewed 16 June 2017>.

what changes could be expected in the years to come. There was also extensive questioning about the amounts of funding needed by the thalidomiders.[332] All in all, this event and the passage of the bill increasing payments to beneficiaries of the German Foundation marked the beginning of serious, politically supported activity to improve the conditions of thalidomide survivors there.

Again, though, it was clear to most campaigners that this was not enough, and so they upped the pressure still further. The heart of activity was in North Rhine Westphalia where about one third of all German Contergan survivors live, and which is also the home state of the Grünenthal company. But by the summer of 2008, there were also many other people not only there but all over Germany actively working in many different ways – from hunger strikes to lawsuits – to promote the cause of the thalidomiders. In response, in November 2008, the government announced that in addition to doubling the payments that had taken effect in July (at an additional cost of €31 million per year), a draft bill was being prepared for parliament proposing further financial improvements. In addition, the government indicated that research would be commissioned into the long-term health problems of the thalidomiders, including how health insurance provision for them could be improved. Although it commented that these proposals would not meet all the demands of the campaigners(!), the government's press statement noted that between 1972 and 2007 the federal government had paid out €437.84 million, a vastly greater amount than the DM 110 million originally granted in 1971.[333] Still, there was no mention of the fact that the actual amount earmarked specifically for thalidomiders from the government in 1971 was not DM 110 million, but just DM 50 million. Nor did it mention that, by 2008, the money provided by Grünenthal to the beneficiaries of the German settlement amounted to barely 12% of the total funding of the foundation, with the balance being met by German taxpayers. This stood in stark contrast to Britain, where almost all of the Thalidomide Trust's funds came from the Distillers Company and its legal successors.

These improvements in funding from the federal government and promises of research to determine future needs and policy were soon

[332] From transcript of Bundestag Parliamentary Committee meeting, Berlin 28 May 2008.

[333] 'Bis zu 9.500 Euro mehr im Jahr – deutliche Verbesserungen für Contergangeschädigte erreicht', press release from Falk/Humme of CDU/CSU Bundestag Fraktion, 13 November 2008, *https://www.cducsu.de/presse/pressemitteilungen/bis-zu-9500-euro-mehr-im-jahr-deutliche-verbesserungen-fuer-contergangeschaedigte-erreicht* <viewed 22 October 2017>.

followed by organisational changes and initiatives. In March 2009, for instance, a reform of the German Contergan Foundation was announced, with the board reduced to seven members, of whom two were to be elected from among the German Contergan survivors. At the same time, it was announced that the foundation would begin considering new claims from people who believed they had been damaged by thalidomide. A year and a half later, on 27 November 2010, Barbara Steffens, Health Minister in the government of North Rhine Westphalia, announced a grant to help the state's Contergan Society to open its own 'Peer to Peer' welfare service, to support the health and welfare needs of the 800 or so thalidomiders living there.[334] Again, there was an international learning dimension here: it was to be based on the UK experience of the HealthLink and Volunteer Visitor services that had been implemented by the Thalidomide Trust three years earlier. This was the first properly designed attempt to assess and meet the physical and psychological challenges encountered by the survivors who were located in Germany. It also created a hub for gathering information and evidence about the true situation of thalidomide victims in Germany. Additional research was carried out at Heidelberg University during 2011 and 2012 in the context of a major project to review the health conditions and life circumstances of 900 thalidomiders in 'the German speaking world'.[335] At about the same time the German Foundation commissioned the international law firm DLA Piper to carry out a comparative survey of the thalidomide compensation payments and disability benefits available to thalidomiders in countries outside Germany, a report that was published in January 2012.[336]

The findings of all this research showed how badly the German thalidomiders were faring both in health outcomes and in financial terms. In light of this, it came as a welcome surprise to many when in February 2013 the government announced that the level of benefits awarded to the German Contergan Foundation was to be increased by a further €120 million per annum starting later that year. This enabled dramatic increases in funding for all the people supported by the

334 *http://www.contergan-nrw.eu/archiv_int_con_thali_konferenz_27_11_2010.htm* <viewed 30 April 2015>.

335 'CONTERGAN: Wiederholt durchzuführende Befragungen zu Problemen, speziellen. Bedarfen und Versorgungsdefiziten von contergangeschädigten Menschen.' Zusammenfassender Bericht über die ersten Untersuchungsergebnisse und Ableitung erster Handlungsempfehlungen Institut für Gerontologie Universität Heidelberg (31 Mai 2012).

336 DLA Piper survey; report for the Conterganstiftung, January 2012.

foundation, with payments for the most severely injured rising to €6,912 per month – up from just €545 just over five years earlier, and a significant increase too on the maximum stipend of €1,152 per month that prevailed between July 2008 and 2013. The new, drastically improved level of payments took effect just six years after the most recent 2007 vigil at Stolberg. German survivors were ecstatic:

> *Really good news – we have got the first numbers for the pension ... We had a lot of talks last week and now they will try to get the Conterganstiftungs-law through in March/April 13 – we will get the pension paid back from the first of Jan. 13 and ... the highest pension will be 6912€ per month ... It is incredible and we still cannot believe it, but it is true – all the tv stations and the newspapers write about it today! We heard the sum before, but – to be honest – we did not believe it first!!!*
>
> *So good night – we will try to sleep though we are quite moved and excited!!!*[337]

All in all, these increases amounted to a total additional funding commitment for the German federal government in excess of €3 billion at 2013 prices over the lifetime of the survivors. More than 50 years after the withdrawal of thalidomide from sale in Germany, benefits to German victims of the tragedy were finally approaching those already in place – often for some time – in Britain. That Chemie Grünenthal's contribution to the settlement remained miniscule, coupled with its refusal to apologise for the catastrophe, however, left a lingering sour taste in spite of the sweetness of this major victory. We will return to the campaign against the firm later in the chapter. Just now, we look at the progress of the UK campaign – inspired to some degree by the successes of the German one – to gain additional funding, and an apology, from the government. After all, Britain's government had made only minor contributions to the Thalidomide Trust, contributions which had been more than offset by taxation, as we have seen.

IN PARLIAMENT

Following the changes to funding, benefits and organisation undertaken by the German federal and state government starting in 2008, UK campaigners soon turned their attention to the question of

[337] Email from Claudia Schmidt-Herterich to Martin Johnson and others, 23 February 2013.

the responsibility of the British government for the catastrophe that had unfolded under its watch. In this, members of the original *Sunday Times* Insight Team who had worked on the story over 30 years earlier came to their aid once again. One former member of the team, journalist Bruce Page, unearthed a report indicating that the British government had been warned in 1957 by the World Health Organisation that the lack of pharmaceutical regulation in Britain coupled with the proliferation of new pharmaceutical companies which did not operate to the standards of the longer-established ones meant that Britain was at risk of a pharmaceutical disaster.[338] This discovery and up-to-date evidence of the rapid physical deterioration experienced by many thalidomiders were then used to brief MPs in a vigorous but low-key parliamentary campaign that ran through most of 2009. The first initiatives were rebuffed by the government – by Health Minister Dawn Primarolo, who had been the junior minister in the Treasury in 2002 when the campaign to abolish the income tax on trust payments had begun. She was now backed in this by Alan Johnson as Secretary of State for Health.[339] Things did not look promising, but the campaigners kept building up their lobbying activity until they had a considerable level of support from backbench MPs.

Then, in June 2009, came a surprise government reshuffle. Alan Johnson was replaced by Andy Burnham, and Dawn Primarolo by Mike O'Brien. Within weeks, it was clear that the Health Ministry's new regime would ensure that the government would now support helping the UK survivors. By December, an agreement was reached. For many UK thalidomiders, the moment when Mike O'Brien stood up in parliament on 17 January 2010 was one of the great events of their lives; not only did they hear a formal expression of regret by the government for all that had happened to them, they also heard that the government would now start contributing to their annual payments.

> *The Government wish to express their sincere regret and deep sympathy for the injury and suffering by all those affected when expectant mothers took the thalidomide drug between 1958 and 1961. We acknowledge both the physical hardship and the*

338 'Thalidomide: Opening the last Chinese Box', unpublished paper by Bruce Page 30/05/09 supplied to MPs and ministers in UK parliament during 2009 by the Thalidomide Trust.

339 Letter to Geoff Adams-Spink (Chairman, Thalidomide Trust National Advisory Council) from Rt Hon Alan Johnson MP Secretary of State for Health, 2 April 2009, stating his strong disagreement with the Thalidomide campaign.

> *emotional difficulties that have faced the children affected and their families as a result of this drug and the challenges that many continue to endure, often on a daily basis. In the light of what happened, a complete review of the machinery for marketing, testing and regulating drugs was initiated, including the enactment of the Medicines Act 1968, which introduced further testing for medicines prior to licensing to ensure that they met acceptable standards of safety and efficacy.*[340]

In what was described as a 'Health Grant', and together with contributions from the governments of Scotland, Wales and Northern Ireland, the UK government pledged £26 million for the 'pilot project' for the first three years. This immediately increased the funds available each year to all UK Thalidomide Trust beneficiaries by 75%. What is more, underpinned by the findings of additional research gathered between 2010 and 2012, a further short but forceful parliamentary campaign in 2012 resulted in a pledge of continuation of funding for at least 10 more years, amounting to an additional £104 million. Moreover, this was accompanied by a promise to continue this level of payments for the lifetimes of the beneficiaries. The combination of extra Diageo funding and substantial government contributions in effect tripled the resources available for UK thalidomiders with immediate effect, and represented combined future commitments in excess of £300 million. The general feeling was that while what they received still fell well short of 21st-century personal injury compensation awards, British thalidomide survivors were finally going to be able to cope with most of their most pressing needs, and furthermore could do so for the rest of their lives.[341]

BREAKTHROUGHS ALL AROUND THE WORLD OF THALIDOMIDE

The years after 2008 also produced several new funding agreements in other countries. In Brazil, for example, the federal court in Sao Paulo ruled on 17 July 2009 that the government had acted with negligence and irresponsibility and should therefore pay out the equivalent of US $45 million to the 600 or so registered thalidomide survivors (from the

[340] The Minister of State, Department of Health (Mr. Mike O'Brien), *Hansard* Vol 503 No. 24 cols. 859-860.

[341] 'Looking to the Future: Evaluation of the Health Grant to Thalidomide-Impaired People', July 2012, Firefly Research and Evaluation Ltd., pp. 7-11, 51-52.

1960s onwards). The award entailed compensation levels of about 100 times what the victims had previously received.[342]

Moreover, six weeks after the Brazilian announcement, a lawsuit was filed against the Belgian government by 118 thalidomide survivors there claiming €65 million.[343] About the same time (September 2009), the Austrian government announced a new scheme to support thalidomiders in that country, establishing a fund of up to €2.8 million.[344] Around 40 additional people were in the process of applying to be recognised in Austria as thalidomide victims, in addition to the eight formerly registered in Austria under the German scheme. By March 2010 the Austrian authorities had identified 66 thalidomide survivors in their country.

Not long afterwards, in January 2010, there was good news from Sweden too, and in this case there were payouts both from the company behind the disaster and the government. As Bjorn Håkansson, the leader of the Swedish Thalidomide Society (FfdN), reported:

> *We have now won a small victory against AstraZeneca. They paid out approx. £10 million to 105 survivors in December, and increased our yearly compensation with 50 percent starting this year, all tax free – but the average payment per year is still low, and for the worst cases around £22,000. We got a lump sum from the Swedish government 2005, it was approx. £45,000 and was paid out to everyone tax free.*[345]

In Ireland, too, the government announced in April 2010 that it was in discussion with 31 thalidomide survivors there about increased funding.[346] Unfortunately, in the view of the Irish thalidomiders, the sum on offer came nowhere near to meeting their needs, so they did not accept the proposals, and settlements remained outstanding through 2014 both there and in Belgium. In Australia, however, a deal was struck in 2010 with Diageo plc and the 45 thalidomide survivors there who had settled with Distillers decades earlier, providing ongoing

342 *http://www.jamaicaobserver.com/magazines/allwoman/155746_Brazil-ordered-to-compensate-thalidomide-victims* <viewed 11 October 2014>.

343 *http://www.spiegel.de/panorama/justiz/belgien-contergan-opfer-fordern-65-millionen-euro-schadensersatz-a-715137.html* <viewed 11 October 2014>.

344 Email from Shoshana Duizend-Jensen, leader of Contergan Austria to Martin Johnson; 16 February 2010.

345 Email from Bjorn Håkansson, President of FfdN to Martin Johnson; 20 January 2010.

346 *http://health.gov.ie/blog/press-release/minister-harney-announces-new-supports-for-survivors-of-thalidomide* <viewed 11 October 2014>.

support on a basis that closely matched the UK funding and valued at £25 million. In December 2013, there was further news from Australia that a settlement of a lawsuit valued at £52 million had been agreed with Diageo plc to support an additional 102 thalidomide victims newly identified there.[347]

The breakthrough in Italy came even earlier, in February 2008, although there had been absolutely nothing available to victims there until that point. Finally, though, and to the great benefit of Italian thalidomiders, the government enacted a law that extended the benefits already accorded to victims of compulsory vaccinations to 250 thalidomide survivors born between 1959 and 1965, the period during which the drug was sold in Italy.[348] This was a far more generous response than that of the Spanish government (mentioned earlier), which started taking action later in 2008, although hardly substantial in comparison to the other countries we have examined in this chapter.

Three shots to the head? Gunning for Grünenthal

We return to the Stolberg vigil of October 2007, which was held at the site of Chemie Grünenthal, the company that had unleashed the thalidomide catastrophe and which was the ultimate target of campaigners. The vigil was one of several events that autumn that placed the German family firm under renewed and sustained pressure. A week before the Stolberg event took place, the company got its first warning of threats from a new quarter when the *Financial Times Magazine* published a nine-page feature article, 'Thalidomide: it's not over yet!' It told the story of the original campaigns for justice in the UK and Germany, and how a 'new wave of campaigns' had now begun. It described the success of the UK thalidomiders in achieving a major improvement to the funding of the Thalidomide Trust in 2005, then valued at £168 million, a sum which represented effectively double the funds previously available. The article also reported on the subsequent determination of the UK campaigners to bring Grünenthal to account

[347] *http://www.theaustralian.com.au/news/nation/thalidomide-victim-lynette-rowe-compensated-for-life-after-distributor-settlement/story-e6frg6nf-1226429113527?nk=0acbb97e2ad1b832a1d80ce868473a9d* <viewed 11 October 2014>; *http://www.theguardian.com/society/2014/feb/07/thalidomide-victims-receive-89m-compensation* <viewed 11 October 2014>. For the Australian story, including information on the lawsuit, see Michael Magazanik, *Silent Shock: The men behind the thalidomide scandal and an Australian family's long road to justice* (Melbourne: Text Publishing, 2015).

[348] DLA Piper survey; report for the Conterganstiftung, January 2012, pp. 93-95.

for what had happened. It also told of Grünenthal CEO Sebastian Wirtz's determination to resist them. Finally, the prominent British campaigner Nick Dobrik was quoted in the *FT* saying:

> *This is going to be a nasty, horrible campaign which could take three or four years with dramatic tactics. With Diageo we just had to put the pistol on the table. With Grünenthal, we'll have to shoot them three times in the head first.*[349]

Increasing pressure from ever more determined campaigners was not the only thorn in the side of Chemie Grünenthal's managers in autumn 2007, though; there were also financial problems. The same day that the *FT* article was published in Britain, an article appeared in the *Financial Times Deutschland* entitled 'Hard Times for Grünenthal'.[350] The piece highlighted the company's slow growth over the previous decade, and noted that Sebastian Wirtz, the CEO since 2005, was hoping to return to more rapid growth by 2009. It also reported on the reaction of the firm to unwanted media attention surrounding a new film, 'Ein einzige Tablette' ('Just a single tablet'), a docu-drama about the Contergan disaster. It was scheduled to be broadcast in November 2007. Wirtz said that his company would prepare employees, 'particularly the sales force, for new questions arising after the transmission of the film'.[351]

In spite of Grünenthal's legal attempts to block the broadcast, which had been ongoing for a year, it was in fact shown on German television on 7 November 2007. The impact was tremendous, and it was every bit as bad a public relations headache for the firm as Wirtz had anticipated: as a docu-drama it told the story in a way that highlighted the impact of the disaster on the families and children affected, and it also portrayed the company in a very poor light. The reaction from Grünenthal was very defensive. In an article published three days after the broadcast, Sebastian Wirtz was cited as saying that his family and the firm did not bear any moral blame for the catastrophe, although they did have a moral responsibility. He tried to justify the company's legal battle to prevent it being shown, in the process indicating that he was 'extremely sorry' that the catastrophe had happened. Here, he was seen to have

349 Andrew Jack, 'Thalidomide: It's Not Over Yet', *Financial Times Magazine* (22/23 September 2007).
350 Peter Kuchenbuch, 'Grünenthal vor Durststrecke', *Financial Times Deutschland* (22 September 2007).
351 *Ibid.*

departed from the previous hard line of resistance to any criticism adopted by his father Michael Wirtz and grandfather Hermann. The article, however, contrasted the position of his company towards German survivors with that of Diageo towards the UK survivors, noting that the British-based multinational had agreed to provide substantial additional funding as recently as 2005.[352]

Remember, too, that ICTA was established in early 2008, specifically targeting Chemie Grünenthal as the ultimate culprit in the thalidomide catastrophe. The combined effect of all of these pressures – and in particular the establishment of ICTA as an activist organisation and the *FT* article – seems to have caused a sense of humour failure in Stolberg, in particular in relation to Nick Dobrik's comments in the *FT* piece; in March 2008 Sebastian Wirtz told a reporter, 'It is not acceptable for individual ICTA members to threaten head shots.'[353] Some campaigners thought it wonderfully ironic that Wirtz was complaining about being 'threatened' with an attack using small arms by a man with – small arms! In any event, the widespread and international media coverage Wirtz's bizarre statement attracted stood the campaign in good stead.

Still waiting for justice

As a result of the combination of vigorous campaigning, new lawsuits and political pressure that got underway in 2005 and gathered in force over the next eight years, the governments of Germany, the UK, Italy, Austria, Spain and Canada, together with the companies that were the legal successors to Astra and Distillers, the key licensees of thalidomide, committed themselves by 2015 to considerable additional future funding for thalidomide survivors. In the latest new settlement in this group announced in 2015, the Canadian government confirmed a total fund of CA $180 million for their 92 eligible survivors.[354] The total new funds available in all of the countries involved in these settlements amounted to the order of several billion pounds, and the

352 'Grünenthal steht bereit, Opfer zu treffen', *Eifeler Nachrichten* / e / Page 1, Saturday, 10 November 2007.

353 Yvonne Esterhazy and Jürgen Salz, 'Britisches Contergan-Opfer fordert von Grünenthal mehr Geld', *Wirtschaftswoche* (30 March 2008): *http://www.wiwo.de/unternehmen/pharma-britisches-contergan-opfer-fordert-von-gruenenthal-mehr-geld/5366362.html* <viewed 22 October 2017>.

354 Statement from Minister Ambrose on Thalidomide, 22nd May 2015: *http://news.gc.ca/web/article-en.do?nid=978709* <viewed 16 October 2015>.

new money worked wonders. It brought dramatic improvements to the lives of some 4,500 thalidomide survivors worldwide, including some 700 who had previously received no compensation whatsoever.[355]

But it is perhaps ironic that this additional funding represented a sum of the same order of magnitude as the valuation in 2006 of Chemie Grünenthal GmbH itself,[356] the company that caused all this disaster in the first place and which is conspicuous by its absence from any of the schemes just described. In other words, apart from its paltry commitment in the early 1970s to provide compensation to German victims only, and its 2008 offer to provide a top-up to this of approximately the same paltry sum that it had previously offered, the firm has managed to evade its responsibility for thalidomide completely.

As a result of the pressure just described, however, the firm did agree in 2008 to a round of discussions with the ICTA leadership, which, perhaps unsurprisingly, turned out to be fruitless once again. But elsewhere things were changing. In Australia, on 13 July 2012 Grünenthal was named as first defendant in a claim prepared by Gordon Legal on behalf of Lynette Rowe, who would be the first of more than 100 claimants in this class action suit.[357] While the successful claimants in this series of legal actions did achieve a settlement with Diageo plc (who represented the other two defendants in the suit, the original Distillers companies) and not Chemie Grünenthal, the outcome signalled that Grünenthal could not rest easy any longer. The Australian action was soon followed by another lawsuit in the USA in October 2012, where a claim was filed in Philadelphia on behalf of 11 people for thalidomide damage.[358]

As had been the case in 2007/8, there were other threats on the horizon for the firm. For one thing, Grünenthal continued to struggle financially; on 9 November 2010, an Aachen newspaper reported that the company had announced major job cuts, affecting about 450 employees by the end of 2013, mainly at the local headquarters and

355 Approximate numbers: 2,750 German settlement, 600 Brazil, 470 UK, 250 Italy, 150 Australia, 100 Astra/Swedish settlement, 90 Canada, 50 Austria, 30 Spain. New beneficiaries: 250 German scheme, 250 Italy, 100 Australia, 100 Austria+Spain+UK.

356 From report on Grünenthal GmbH supplied to the Thalidomide Trust by Schroder Investment Management Ltd, 12 May 2006, including reports from Dunn & Bradstreet and Bureau van Dijk.

357 Supreme Court of Victoria at Melbourne, reference SCI 2011 3527 dated 13 July 2012. For a full account of the preparations for and conduct of the lawsuit by one of the lawyers in this team, see Michael Magazanik, *Silent Shock*.

358 *http://www.post-gazette.com/news/health/2012/10/22/Thalidomide-s-uneasy-return/stories/201210220238* <viewed 11 October 2014>.

production site. As a result, the original factory at Stolberg where Contergan was manufactured would be closed. Through this, it was hoped to achieve annual savings of €57 million. The plan was to reinvest some of the savings into the company's activities in the USA and Brazil.[359] Whether this was a retrenchment of the business or an attempt to move the main business activities of the firm away from the thalidomide risks is not clear. The company certainly placed most of its hopes for a business turnaround on a potential takeover by the giant American pharmaceutical company, Johnson & Johnson, which had been signalled by the American-based firm's Harald Stock replacing Sebastian Wirtz as CEO in 2008. Stock was the first non-family member to take charge of the company.[360]

In the meantime, no doubt because the company continued to be under serious pressure on a number of fronts, key Grünenthal staff took part in a series of meetings with a small group of British thalidomide activists during 2013.[361] In this, the company's representatives hoped to persuade the group that access to a separate fund they had recently established to provide a maximum of €3,000 for equipment for 'hardship' cases would satisfy the needs of the thalidomide community.[362] The thalidomiders felt this approach would be unsatisfactory in spite of the firm's characterisation of the offer by May 2013 as a 'Social Inclusion' project. A senior Grünenthal delegate also disclosed to the campaigners that there was serious disagreement among the family shareholders, with some of the younger ones wanting to find a way of resolving the thalidomide legacy while the older ones felt they should stand firm. The company's representative also confirmed that the hope of selling the company to Johnson & Johnson was now at an end, and the departure of Harald Stock as CEO in May 2013 confirmed that.[363]

359 *http://www.aachener-nachrichten.de/lokales/stolberg/gruenenthal-baut-weltweit-360-stellen-ab-1.365702* <viewed 11 October 2014>.

360 Grünenthal findet neuer chief, in *Manager Magazin* (18 November 2008): *http://www.manager-magazin.de/unternehmen/karriere/a-591240.html* <viewed 13 October 2014>.

361 Letter to Rt. Hon. Michael Moore MP from Harald Stock, CEO Grünenthal, 8 April 2013 re. Grünenthal meetings attended by Stevie Sinclair.

362 Email from Claudia Schmidt-Herterich to Martin Johnson; 2 May 2015.

363 Reports by Stevie Sinclair (Thalidomide UK member) to Martin Johnson 24 May 2013; 21st February 2014. On Stock's departure, see: *https://www.grunenthal.co.uk/cms/cda/file/pm_2013_29_05_Reorganization+of+the+Corporate+Management+structure+of+Gr%C3%BCnenthal+Group_EN.pdf?fileID=255300053&cacheFix=1369810641000&__k=7b8a5d423e4aeb8ac76077a865da4132* <viewed 11 October 2014>. The relationship between the German firm and the American giant came as a result of licensing agreements for drugs to Johnson &

The combination of pressure from campaigners, financial difficulties and differences of opinion within the Wirtz family, apparently along generational lines, may have formed the background to Grünenthal's first public 'apology' – it was, in fact, merely an expression of regret, in spite of some press reports – for the thalidomide disaster, which was delivered by Harald Stock on 31 August 2012.[364] The worldwide rejection of this 'apology' was encapsulated in a Reuters blog article written by Sir Harold Evans and published on 12 September 2012 under the title 'Thalidomide's big lie overshadows corporate apology'.[365] For Evans, the big lie lay in the fact that the company continued to assert that 'Grünenthal acted in accordance with the state of scientific knowledge and all industry standards for testing new drugs that were relevant and acknowledged in the 1950s and 1960s',[366] when in fact that was most certainly not the case.

More seriously for the company, however, it lost a thalidomide lawsuit for the very first time. This was in Spain, where legal action had been brought by Avite, an association representing 180 Spanish thalidomiders. It sought compensation of €204 million for its members. In a ruling dated 21 November 2013, the court found against Grünenthal and ruled that it should 'compensate each one of the plaintiffs' to the tune of tens of thousands of euros each depending on the severity of their disability and also pay legal costs.[367] Sadly, the victory was short-lived: in October 2014, a Spanish Court of Appeals ruled that the claims were to be disallowed as they were 'out of date', i.e. beyond the statute of limitations. The same principle formed the basis for the dismissal of the class action suit in the United States. On 17 October 2014 in Philadelphia, the presiding judge ruled that the claim of damage from thalidomide concerned injuries that were sustained at a time that was beyond the statute of limitations, thus

Johnson and its Janssen subsidiary: *http://www.grunenthal.com/cms/cda/file/2010-06-07_Licensing+Agreement+Tapentadol.pdf?fileID=134500017&cacheFix=1279095184000&_k=87ff3152d40875f5b8456849443294d0* <viewed 11 October 2014>.

364 *http://www.telegraph.co.uk/health/healthnews/9513858/Grunenthals-thalidomide-apology-in-full.html* <viewed 11 October 2011>.

365 *http://blogs.reuters.com/great-debate/2012/09/12/thalidomides-big-lie-overshadows-corporate-apology* <viewed 11 October 2012>.

366 *http://www.telegraph.co.uk/health/healthnews/9513858/Grunenthals-thalidomide-apology-in-full.html* <viewed 11 October 2011>.

367 *http://www.internationallawoffice.com/newsletters/detail.aspx?g=bcec23f0-6c9e-433d-9701-2a48fa6a266e* <viewed 11 October 2014>; *http://www.abc.es/gestordocumental/uploads/Sociedad/Sentencia%20Juzgado%20Primera%20Instancia%2090%20(Caso%20TALIDOMIDA).pdf* <viewed 11 October 2014>.

ending any serious hopes of achieving a new set of thalidomide settlements in the USA.[368]

Nevertheless, 2014 brought some hopeful news to those engaged in the elusive quest for justice in holding Chemie Grünenthal to account for its crimes, even if the ultimate outcome has, as in the case of the lawsuits in Spain and the USA, been ultimately extremely disappointing. On 4 February 2014, the Health Minister of North Rhine Westphalia (NRW) announced she was commissioning an independent inquiry by the Westphälische Wilhelm University in Münster into the state government's conduct in regard to the thalidomide trial that ended, as we saw in Chapter 6, without a conviction.[369] Finally, it appeared that there would be a full-scale investigation into allegations of possible collusion and corruption by the NRW state authorities that had been aired first by Gero Gemballa in 1993 in his book *Der dreifache Skandal* (*The threefold scandal*) where he pointed to the obvious conflict of interest that arose when Dr. Josef Neuberger, the defence attorney for some of the main defendants in the German thalidomide trial to that point, took up the post of Justice Minister for NRW on 8 December 1966.[370] As we have seen in Chapter 6, Neuberger stepped aside as defence attorney, but retained his partnership in and contacts with his law firm, which continued to represent the accused Grünenthal managers throughout the trial. As Justice Minister, of course, Neuberger ultimately oversaw the public prosecutor's office in its handling of the case and also played a role in appointing the judges who oversaw it. The report commissioned by the state of NRW has since appeared, however, and although it provides extensive evidence to support our assessment of the improprieties in the conduct of the Contergan trial presented in Chapter 6, it nevertheless draws the remarkable and baffling conclusion that there were no such improprieties.[371]

368 *http://www.thelegalintelligencer.com/id=1202673704974/Eastern-District-Judge-Tosses-Thalidomide-Case-Against-GSK?slreturn=20150401091201#ixzz3GO17RXR0* <viewed 1 May 2015>.

369 *http://www.mgepa.nrw.de/ministerium/presse/pressemitteilungsarchiv/pm2014/pm20140128a/index.php* <viewed 1 May 2015>. The PhD cum official report has now appeared as: Niklas Lenhard-Schramm, 'Die Haltung des Landes Nordrhein-Westfalen zu Contergan und den Folgen,' PhD dissertation, University of Münster, 2016.

370 Gero Gemballa, *Der dreifache Skandal; 30 Jahre nach Contergan. Eine Dokumentation* (Hamburg: Luchterhand Literaturverlag, 1993) pp. 67-68.

371 Lenhard-Schramm, 'Die Haltung', e.g. pp. 656, 659-661.

Meanwhile, in London, at about the same time the report was commissioned by the state of NRW, the British campaign group decided to approach the German federal government to ask for assistance in seeking compensation from Grünenthal. But the British campaigners also asserted that the German federal government itself had a responsibility to all non-German thalidomide survivors which it had evaded for years owing to the stipulations of the parliamentary act from 1972 creating the German foundation. This legislation and subsequent additions to it had the practical effect of banning thalidomide claims from most non-German nationals in spite of the fact that in most cases the drug had been produced in Germany by Grünenthal and sold in places like Belgium, Italy and Spain by licensed distributors.[372] What is more, the campaigners pointed to German governmental culpability for the longstanding physical and financial plight of both German and non-German survivors owing to its role in bringing the trial of Grünenthal executives to an inconclusive end.

To gain the attention of the German authorities, campaigners approached British MPs for support and also made contact with the European Parliament and the European Commission. However, the response received by Neil Parish MP in April 2014 from German Health Minister Elke Ferner made it plain that she did not consider her government responsible in any way, asserting furthermore that the federal government had no role whatsoever in the termination of the trial of Grünenthal in 1970:

> *...the Federal Government of the time never influenced the trial against Grünenthal. The constitutional principle of the division of power between the legislative, the executive and the judiciary precludes any action aimed at influencing ongoing legal proceedings and guarantees the independence of the judiciary. Accordingly, the decision to suspend proceedings against Grünenthal rested solely with the regional court that had jurisdiction at the time, the Landgericht Aachen, with the consent of the public prosecutor's office ... Nor has any German Federal Government ever intervened in any other way to protect the company...*[373]

372 *Bundesgesetzblatt,* Jahrgang 1971, Teil 1; Gesetz über die Errichtung einer Stiftung, Hilfswerk für behinderte Kinder‘; vom 17 Dezember 1971.

373 Letter from Elke Ferner Parliamentarische Staatssekretärin im BMFSFJ to Mr. Neil Parish MP dated Berlin, 8 April 2014.

As we have seen in Chapter 6, however, this assertion of non-involvement by the German federal authorities in the ending of the trial is certainly not true, as confirmed by evidence from a large number of archival documents compiled in 2014-2015 by one of the authors, Tobias Arndt, who was working in conjunction with the Thalidomide Trust and campaigners. The British group in turn asked a leading international law firm, Ince & Co., for a formal legal opinion on the significance of the documentary evidence. Part of the reply said:

> *Along with our colleagues in Germany, we have examined the documents produced to us and can confirm the contents are as follows, with comment as appropriate:-*
>
> *Federal Health Ministry file note dated 21 July 1969 records a secret (confidentiality was sought by Grünenthal) meeting between Grünenthal directors, including Wirtz a principal defendant in the criminal trial, their lawyers and the Health Ministry at which settlement of the claims was discussed. No victims nor their representatives were involved nor advised of this meeting.*
>
> *Federal Health Ministry file note dated 18 September 1969 records follow up actions and notes discussions between the Federal Health Ministry, the Federal Ministry for Internal Affairs and the Federal Ministry of Labour and Social Affairs (who also wanted the Federal Ministry of Economics and the Federal Ministry of Finance to be involved). The Ministries agreed that a political level discussion was required.*
>
> *Federal Health Ministry file note dated 18 September 1969 (sequel) notes that a solution had to be discussed at a higher level. The Health Ministry was aware that such negotiations could be interpreted as an attempt to interfere with the ongoing criminal trial and should be postponed until after the trial. Nevertheless the German settlement and legislative process continued and was announced publicly in April 1970 despite the fact that the trial was continuing and was not terminated until December 1970.*[374]

In the view of the lawyers from Ince & Co., these and additional

[374] Letter from Ince & Co to the National Advisory Council of the Thalidomide Trust, dated 29 August 2014.

points demonstrate that there is a *prima facie* case to answer about the role of the Germen federal government in the premature suspension of the trial on terms that were grossly inadequate for the victims of Grünenthal. But the larger significance of this intervention is easily missed and even more troubling. After all, it was not the role of this trial to award compensation to the surviving victims of the company in personal injury matters, but instead to determine the guilt or innocence of those charged with carrying out an enormous and monstrous crime. To terminate the proceedings without a verdict left the profound issue of responsibility for this crime unresolved. The fact that the trial was brought to a premature end on the basis of a woefully inadequate settlement – and under terms that protected the company that produced this diabolical drug and its managers – made things even worse.

These are the issues that the British campaigners, now in conjunction with other thalidomide groups from Europe and across the world, are determined to tackle once and for all. Their first target is the organisation which appears to have done the most to bring about this cover-up and colossal miscarriage of justice, the German federal government, and by the end of 2016 they were making progress. An intensive lobbying campaign in the European Parliament by thalidomiders from across Europe resulted in a unanimous resolution calling upon the German government to provide support for 'all EU citizens affected by Thalidomide' on 15 December 2016.[375] The unanimous resolution was a remarkable political achievement, and it also contained an amendment calling on Grünenthal to be required to provide compensation and care, which was passed separately by a considerable majority. Although the resolution was non-binding, it put pressure on the German government to take action in support of the surviving victims of thalidomide.

Still, the black balloons seen in Stolberg and London that commemorate the vast number of thalidomide children who died point to the continuing need for justice for them too, not just from the German government, but more importantly from the company that perpetrated the crime. Only when Chemie Grünenthal is finally held to account for the vast toll of death and injuries caused by their drug will the quest for justice be complete.

[375] EU Parliament press release, 15 December 2016: *http://www.europarl.europa.eu/news/en/news-room/20161208IPR55202/meps-call-for-better-access-to-compensation-for-thalidomide-victims* <viewed 20 December 2016>.

Figure 13: Thalidomide catastrophe timeline.

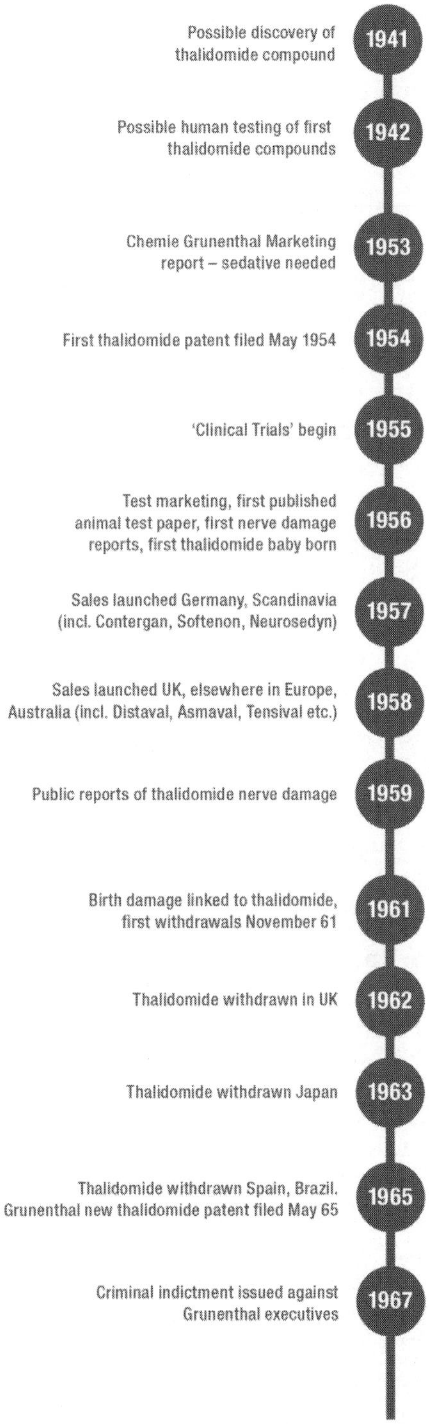

- **1968** Criminal trial of Grunenthal executives begins
- **1969** Swedish settlement agreed by Astra company
- **1970** Trial closed Germany December 1970
- **1971** German Foundation law enacted
- **1972** German thalidomide foundation established
- **1973** Settlement agreed UK
- **1974** UK Thalidomide Trust and Japanese Ishizue foundation formed
- **1975** Brazil Leprosy-related thalidomide births begin
- **2007** Spanish government finally agrees thalidomide distributed in Spain. Most recent thalidomide patent filed by scientists connected to Grunenthal
- **2008** German foundation doubles payments to thalidomiders; Italian government announces new funding scheme for thalidomiders
- **2009** Brazilian government announces increases thalidomide payments up to 100 fold, Austrian government announces new scheme funding thalidomiders
- **2010** British government apology for thalidomide, new govt. funding for UK thalidomiders; Spanish government compensation scheme established; new funding scheme for Scandinavian thalidomiders; thalidomide child born in Brazil; new Diageo funding scheme for 45 Australian thalidomiders
- **2012** New settlement announced for another 102 Australian thalidomiders
- **2015** Canadian government announces new funding scheme for Canadian thalidomiders

CHAPTER EIGHT

Thalidomide – from 1961 to the Present

The never-ending human experiment.

ANY REASONABLE PERSON WOULD ASSUME that because of the thalidomide catastrophe, Grünenthal would have abandoned all interest in producing or selling the drug after its withdrawal from sale in November 1961. Certainly, the other main companies involved all did so. In the UK, for example, the reaction of the Distillers Company was to withdraw from pharmaceuticals completely, and the company sold the division that had marketed thalidomide to Eli Lilley. Astra, the Scandinavian company, abandoned thalidomide, too, as did Richardson Merrell in the USA (where it had not been licensed by the Food and Drug Administration for sale) and Canada (where it had been licensed for sale). A number of smaller licensee companies in Italy went bankrupt.

But Grünenthal was different. In fact, evidence from patents demonstrates clearly that research and development work on thalidomide at the company did not even pause for breath or reflection in the aftermath of the drug's withdrawal from general sale; the first new patent was registered by Grünenthal already in 1965. Between then and 2001, the firm applied for a total of 24 patents covering about 250 thalidomide-like chemicals and related manufacturing processes. (Details are in Appendix 3.) What is more, in contrast to the company's earlier reluctance in 1961 to spend any money on testing for antivitamin risks (which may have revealed a potential teratogenic effect), it invested with gusto in these patents in the form of initial submissions fees in many countries and renewal fees in these and others.

Over the years, the cost of this activity – leaving aside entirely the cost of the R&D necessary to generate these applications – has far exceeded the probable cost of vital testing which should have been undertaken at the outset.[376]

In other words, even while the thalidomide case was being prepared for trial, even while the trial was taking place, even while claims were being made in the courts for thousands of damaged children around the world and even as many parents were still burying their dead thalidomide children, Grünenthal scientists were busily seeking ways to develop and exploit this drug, which had caused the world's worst catastrophe of its kind. Moreover, this activity was directly supervised up until at least 1974 by Dr. Heinrich Mückter, the company's chief scientist, as can be seen from the fact that he was a named inventor on several of the patents that were filed. In fact, he was registered on four thalidomide-type patents filed between October 1965 and 1967, i.e. at the time that he was awaiting trial on criminal charges for his role in the thalidomide catastrophe. (See Appendix 3.) And even after Grünenthal withdrew entirely from the thalidomide market in 2003,[377] another company, the Celgene Division of the Celanese Corporation, which had taken a licence for thalidomide in the United States in the late 1990s,[378] continued to operate in this market.

Why? And with what effects? The first question can be answered with one word – greed – but a fuller answer revolves around the dogged pursuit of what we might now call a 'killer app' for the drug. Initially, from the mid-1960s onwards, treatment of leprosy was the focus. From the 1980s, the target was AIDS, while cancer treatment was the focus from the 1990s onwards. Since then, thalidomide has been touted as an

376 The same applies to the original thalidomide patents from 1954 and 1956. Where documentation on the duration of the patents was available, which was the case for Canada and West Germany, the patents had been extended to the longest possible period into the 1970s. To extend a patent to its longest possible duration is generally quite expensive: Annual extension or renewal fees for patents rise in order to prevent protective patenting and to benefit from profitable intellectual property. In some countries, a renewal for the final year alone can cost as much as the first 5 or even 8 years of a patent protection. One of the co-authors of this book, Tobias Arndt, estimates that the renewals of the original thalidomide patents – if as the two positive findings suggest – applied to all original thalidomide patents to the maximum allowable period would have cost at current tariffs at least €100,000. Also see appendix 1 for the list of identified original thalidomide patents, which is likely not to be complete.

377 In a letter from Grünenthal to Dr. Claes Malm, Haematology Clinic, Linköping, Sweden dated 2003-08-02 Dr. Klaus Wilsmann explains that Grünenthal will cease supplying thalidomide after 15 June 2003 (copy letter held by the authors).

378 Hawthorne F., *Inside the FDA: The Business and Politics Behind the Drugs We Take and the Food We Eat* (NY: John Wiley, 2005) pp. 110-111.

effective treatment of: Alzheimer's disease;[379] lupus and other auto-immune diseases;[380] and even (in the form of a thalidomide derivative) as an elixir to counter the effects of ageing.[381] In every case, the drug has been at best ineffective in treating the target disease or illness, and in fact usually caused harm, particularly in relation to the side effects that we know about already. The answer to the second question, then, is 'with disastrous effects', as we will see in detail shortly. These have involved excruciating and permanent nerve damage among many taking the drug. And, in the case of treatment from 1972 onward for the ENL complication of leprosy in Brazil, another epidemic of thalidomide-induced birth defects occurred: it is estimated at least 1,000 thalidomide children were born there since the early 1970s because their mothers were supplied with the drug as a leprosy-related treatment or because they were given it by someone undergoing such treatment.[382] Killer apps indeed!

Thalidomide and leprosy

How did thalidomide become so widely known in connection with treating leprosy? It began with experiments on leprosy patients that involved a radical change in accepted treatment patterns, which in turn started not long after the withdrawal of thalidomide from general sale. The basic facts are as follows. In 1965, an Israeli doctor, Professor Jacob Sheshkin, reported carrying out a trial the previous year with a group of leprosy patients using thalidomide to treat a complication of the disease called 'Erythema Nodosum Leprosum', or ENL. 'Erythema Nodosum' is a term used more generally to describe a skin inflammation producing painful and tender lumps, usually on the legs. ENL is a specific form of this disorder associated with leprosy in which the inflammation appears all over the body. It is not considered life-threatening and had never been regarded as a high priority problem to be solved because it affected only a very small number of people suffering from leprosy. What changed in the second half of the 20th

[379] Michael Slenske (2012), 'Thalidomide Made Good: One of History's Most Feared and Stigmatized Drugs Re-emerges as a Potential Cure for Alzheimer's'; *Phoenix Magazine,* p. 96.

[380] Salynn Boyles (2012), 'Drug Shows Promise for Lupus Skin Conditions', *WebMD: http://lupus.webmd.com/news/20121205/drug-lupus-skin-conditions* <viewed 7 January 2013>.

[381] *http://www.huffingtonpost.com/arlene-weintraub/could-thalidomide-be-resu_b_797912.html* <viewed 4 January 2012>.

[382] World Health Organisation, Leprosy Team, May 2003, 'No Role for Thalidomide in Leprosy', The Pan American Health Organisation: *http://www.paho.org/English/AD/DPC/CD/thalidomide.htm* <viewed 21 July 2011>.

century, however, was the development of effective drug treatments for leprosy which had the side effect of dramatically increasing the incidence of ENL.[383]

This side effect was particularly pronounced among those taking part in Sheshkin's trial because he was administering the leprosy drug Dapsone to them at the exceptionally high level of 700 mg weekly – 35 times the maximum weekly dose of 20 mg recommended by most specialists at the time. In other words, Sheshkin's patients each week received the amount of medication that would normally be given over the course of nine months. Given that the incidence of ENL in patients tended to be worse with higher Dapsone treatment levels, it is not surprising that Sheshkin's patients experienced ENL at far higher rates than the one in 20 on average that would be expected at normal levels of Dapsone ingestion.

So, he had a problem. But he claimed to have solved it almost immediately by dosing the patients with thalidomide, thus alleviating the symptoms of ENL.[384] Effectively, though, he was trying to fix a problem caused by one pharmaceutical treatment by adding another treatment to the mix, something which admittedly happens frequently in drug therapies. In this case, though, leprosy patients who were suffering a progressive disease of the nervous system were now being put at further risk by having their nervous systems permanently wrecked by damage caused by thalidomide. This was something pointed out in 1994 by Dr. Colin Crawford in a paper demonstrating that many of the researchers using thalidomide to treat ENL either failed to report testing for neuropathic effects of the drug or reported tests of an inappropriate type to reveal thalidomide neuropathy.[385] In other words, the far cheaper and safer course of treatment would have been to reduce the incidence of ENL by reducing the Dapsone dose.

Yet these dangers were largely ignored for a considerable amount of time, not just by Sheshkin, but by other highly influential parties. The World Health Organisation (WHO), for example, reviewed the use of thalidomide for ENL in 1977, but appeared to take no account of the neuropathic risks. By the early 1980s, the drug was being used very widely for this purpose, and in 1988, the WHO expert committee on

383 Sheskin J., 'Thalidomide in the treatment of lepra reactions.', *Clin Pharm Therap* 1965; 6: 303.
384 *Ibid.*
385 Crawford, C.L. (1994) 'Use of Thalidomide in Leprosy', *Adverse Drug and Toxicological Reviews* 13(4):177-192.

leprosy provided guidelines for its use, again omitting mention of neuropathy while at the same time warning that it should only be given to men and post-menopausal women.[386] Soon after that, the news that thalidomide in Brazil was causing birth defects called this policy into question, while Colin Crawford's 1994 paper demonstrated the dangers of nerve damage associated with the drug. Still, nothing was done in the short term; it was only in 2003 that the WHO finally produced a report stating that there is 'No Role for Thalidomide in Leprosy'.[387]

In the meantime, however, Sheshkin and others had been extraordinarily successful in instead attaining a prominent role for thalidomide in leprosy treatment. Already in the very same year as Sheshkin's first published study, 1965, Brazil approved the use of thalidomide for the treatment of ENL.[388] By 1973, a number of other leprosy researchers followed Sheshkin's lead, and a global drive to use thalidomide began. Despite official warnings (that thalidomide should only be used for 'strictly investigative purposes'), it was being used by the early 1970s in at least 62 centres, many in the developing world.[389]

The damage was not long in coming. From the 1990s onwards, a series of studies have reported births of thalidomide children in Latin American countries, mainly Brazil. Birth defect registers and similar monitoring systems cover only a small part of the population concerned, but one study of a total of 1,145,214 births in Brazil between 1982 and 2008 found 261 reports of babies with a probable pattern of thalidomide damage.[390] Brazil is a country with a population in 2010 of 190,000,000 but a high birth rate. It is therefore likely that the estimated number of 1,000 surviving thalidomide children in Brazil vastly understates the true scale of the problem. It is also the case that the rate at which thalidomide children are being born does not appear to have diminished significantly despite the WHO's belated warnings on the subject. An explanation for this phenomenon has been offered by

[386] *Ibid.*

[387] *Ibid,;* World Health Organisation, Leprosy Team, May 2003, 'No Role for Thalidomide in Leprosy', The Pan American Health Organisation: *http://www.paho.org/English/AD/DPC/CD/thalidomide.htm* <viewed 21 July 2011>.

[388] Oliveira M.A., Bermudez J.A.Z., Souza A.C. (1999) 'Talidomida no Brasil: vigilância com responsabilidade compartilhada?', *Cademos de Saúde Pública.* 1999; 15:99-112.

[389] Crawford, C.L. (1994) 'Use of Thalidomide in Leprosy', in *Adverse Drug and Toxicological Reviews* 13(4):183, 1994.

[390] F.S.L. Vianna, J.S. Lopez-Camelo, J.C.L. Leite, M.T.V. Sanseverino, M. de G. Dutra, E.E. Castilla, L. Schuler-Faccini (2011)' Epidemiological Surveillance of Birth Defects Compatible with Thalidomide Embryopathy in Brazil', *PLoS One* 2011; 6(7): e21735 PMCID: PMC3130769.

Dr. Eduardo E. Castilla, author of a number of reports on the rise of thalidomide teratogenicity in Latin America:

> *But, on the contrary, thalidomide is prescribed for years; clearly showing that WHO arguments can not stand a confrontation with hard realities. Obviously, physicians are willing to prescribe thalidomide to patients despite the fact that thalidomide is a well-known human teratogen. In fact, it's not seldom that the patient himself is the driving force in a prescription situation. Thalidomide acts as a tranquilizer. The patient gets addicted to the drug, and wants more, and more.*[391]

In Brazil, the situation was complicated still further by the fact that the drug was prescribed and distributed free of charge to leprosy patients, and it seems to have remained the drug of choice there because of its low cost of production. This means that it is very likely that it would be passed on by the leprosy patients to their (non-leprosy-affected) friends. A report in 2007 on three thalidomide children born in Brazil in 2005 and 2006 noted that 'in two of the three cases the mother was not the person on treatment but used thalidomide by proxy, that is, through the well-recognized popular habit of sharing medications'.[392]

We've looked at the fact that thalidomide was used increasingly as a leprosy treatment, in particular in connection with ENL. And we have seen the devastation that resulted. But what we have not examined is who supplied it. After all, the quantities of thalidomide tablets must have been enormous to wreak such havoc.

Let us start with the source of supplies to the first scientist who reported using thalidomide for ENL, Professor Jacob Sheshkin. Sheshkin was born in Poland and qualified as a doctor in 1940 with degrees from the universities of Vilna (1939) and Kovno (1940). A Jew, he escaped the Holocaust and returned to Poland to teach at Warsaw University in 1945. After teaching in Caracas University (Venezuela)

[391] E.E. Castilla, P. Ashton-Prolla, E. Barreda-Meija, D. Brunoni, D.P. Cavalcanti, J. Correa-Neto, J.L. Degadillo, M.G. Dutra, T. Felix, A. Giraldo, N. Juarez, J.S. Lopez-Camelo, J. Nazer, I.M. Oriolli, J.E. Paz, M. Pesseto, J.M. Pina-Neto, R. Quadrelli, M. Rittler, S. Rueda, M. Saltos, O. Sanchez, L. Schuler (1996) 'Thalidomide, A Current Teratogen in South America', *Teratology* 54:273-277 (1996); and in report published by Föreningen för de Neurosedynskadade, Stockholm at: *http://www.thalidomide.org/web/children-born-i-brazil* <viewed 23 July 2011>.

[392] L. Schuler-Faccini, R.C.F. Soares, A.C.M. de Sousa, C. Maximino, E. Luna, I.V.D. Schwartz, C. Waldman, E.E. Castilla (2007) 'New Cases of Thalidomide Embryopathy in Brazil', *Birth Defects Research (Part A)* 79:671-672 (2007).

and Madrid University, he was appointed to the Hebrew University in Jerusalem in 1956, where he was working at the time he began his experiments with thalidomide.[393] In the papers he published in the 1960s, he did not disclose where he had obtained thalidomide from, nor did he mention any connection with Grünenthal. In 1969, however, he published a paper where he listed 'von Beielstein H.' as co-author.[394] This was Dr. Hans Werner von Schrader Beielstein, Grünenthal's head of marketing, a colleague and close personal friend of Dr. Heinrich Mückter and, at the time the article was published, on trial in Alsdorf along with other Grünenthal top managers for their role in the thalidomide catastrophe. Von Schrader Beielstein had become an employee of Grünenthal in February 1957, initially as the company's Medical Advisor. Shortly before that, in the same year, Heinrich Mückter's former boss from the Kraków Institute during the war, Professor Eyer, had ended von Schrader Beielstein's hopes for an academic career at the University of Bonn by declining to support him for the key qualification (Privatdozent) needed to become a professor. Von Schrader Beielstein subsequently became involved in the foreign licence department and was from September 1961 head of Grünenthal's 'Contergan committee'.

Von Schrader Beielstein's appearance as co-author of the 1969 paper strongly suggests that Sheshkin's supplies of thalidomide came from Grünenthal, which is all the more likely given the fact that for more than 30 years after the end of 1961, there was no company known to produce or distribute thalidomide on anything other than the tiniest scale except for the German firm.

But another paper on treatment of ENL using thalidomide by M. F. R. Waters in 1971 is more explicit about the source of the drug and also ties in directly with Sheshkin, who is cited in the article as the author of six different studies. The paper discusses tests involving ten patients in Malaysia. In the acknowledgements, Waters states, 'Thanks are also due to Dr. H.W. von Schrader Beielstein of Chemie Grünenthal, Stolberg, West Germany, for the supply of both thalidomide and placebo.'[395] In other words, at the very time he was supporting Sheshkin in his unusual leprosy experiments in Israel, and assisting Waters with

393 *http://prof-jakob-sheskin.tripod.com* <viewed 23 July 2011>.

394 Sheshkin J., Sagher F., Dorfraan M., Von Beielstein H., 'Unsatisfactory results with thalidomide as a specific treatment for leprosy.', *Israel J. Med. Sci.* 1968; 4: 901-4.

395 Waters M.F.R. (1971), 'An Internally-controlled Double Blind Trial of Thalidomide in Severe Erythema Nodosum Leprosum', *Leprosy Review* (1971) 42, 26-42.

his research in Malaysia, von Schrader Beielstein was standing trial on criminal charges at Alsdorf.

Crawford's 1994 paper also mentioned Grünenthal explicitly as the source of the drug:

> *By 1973 it was being used in at least 62 centres many of which were in developing countries. By 1974 it had become the drug of choice... for the management of ENL. The drug was obtainable directly from Chemie Grünenthal but WHO set up no advisory body to monitor the side effects, or even to record how many patients were being treated. The widespread use in developing countries created a new danger because of the absence of any statutory body to monitor side effects and because of the frequency with which drugs are stolen and misused.*[396]

Grünenthal did admit in 2003 that it had supplied the drug to a number of researchers and other users over the course of the past four decades or so, but gave the impression that it had done so as a sort of *pro bono* arrangement in the service of science and humanity and that it had long since stopped manufacturing thalidomide:

> *In the last 20 years we were able to help thousands of patients, relatives, and medical institutions by providing thalidomide free of charge. As our reserves have now been exhausted, we are no longer able to provide this aid.*[397]

It is, of course, extremely unlikely that the company was supplying the drug gratis. After all, the large amounts of money the firm spent on R&D and patent activity relating to the drug after 1961 had to come from somewhere. And it is quite simply unbelievable that it would have had reserves on hand from production that occurred through November 1961 that would be sufficient to supply researchers around the world and users in large numbers, mostly in the Third World, for more than forty years after thalidomide's withdrawal from general sale. What is more, there is in fact evidence that Grünenthal *was* manufacturing the drug for treatment of ENL after 1961 in spite of the company's self-serving 2003 statement. Christian Wagemann, a former Grünenthal

[396] Crawford, C.L. (1994), 'Use of Thalidomide in Leprosy', *Adverse Drug and Toxicological Reviews* 13(4):183, 1994.

[397] In a letter from Grünenthal to Dr. Claes Malm, Haematology Clinic, Linköping, Sweden dated 2003-08-02 Dr. Klaus Wilsmann explains that Grünenthal will cease supplying thalidomide after 15th June 2003 (copy letter held by the Thalidomide Trust).

chemist and engineer who began working for the firm in 1973, has said that everyone knew the building that was being used for making thalidomide as well as when it was being produced because of the very distinctive smell of the chemicals involved.[398] And in 1972, the company actually revealed in an interview with a local journalist entitled 'Contergan firm fights leprosy' that it did not give away the drug in order to reduce unsellable stock. In fact, a Grünenthal spokesman insisted that the thalidomide for fighting leprosy was specially manufactured, and he furthermore predicted that thalidomide might possibly be sold commercially by the company again in the very near future.[399]

Thalidomide use with HIV and AIDS

The patents listed in Appendix 3 that were registered between 1994 and 2001 refer to a variety of ulcer conditions, including Behçet's disease, Aphthous ulcers, Pyoderma Gangranosum and orogenital ulcers generally. These references in turn relate to the discovery that thalidomide is allegedly particularly effective at providing rapid relief to this type of condition. It is possible that this discovery was made during the course of leprosy research. But because one of the common side effects of HIV/AIDS is severe ulceration of the whole mouth, right to the pharynx at the back (Aphthous ulcers), with consequent great difficulty in eating and swallowing that contribute to dangerous levels of weight loss, the AIDS epidemic of the 1980s paved the way for treatment with thalidomide. In fact, by the early 1990s, it had been found that thalidomide could bring about a rapid clearing of these ulcers, enabling patients to start eating again.[400]

Whether or not research associated with the ENL treatment regime in Latin America led to the use of thalidomide as a treatment for complications associated with AIDS/HIV in the United States, there was a direct material connection between the two. Thalidomide, which was believed to be helpful in treatment of some of the effects of AIDS, was not available in the US; it was therefore sourced through the black

398 Interview with Christian Wagemann by Monika Eisenberg and Martin Johnson, 7 July 2009, Aachen.

399 'Contergan-Firma Bekämpft Lepra; Chemie Grünenthal verschenkt Thalidomide an bedürftige Länder'; *Ruhr Nachrichten* (18 July 1972).

400 Paterson D.L., Georghiou P.R., Allworth A.M., Kemp R.J. (1995) 'Thalidomide as a Treatment of refractory Aphthous Ulceration Related to Human Immunodeficiency Virus Infection', *Clinical Infectious Diseases*, Vol. 20, No. 2, (February 1995) pp. 250-4.

market, smuggled in from Central and South America, where it was freely available as a result of its use for ENL.

There was yet another link to the ENL story in terms of the effects on those who took thalidomide to alleviate their symptoms. For AIDS patients, too, thalidomide did not in the end prove to be an effective cure for the side effects of their disease in spite of initial high hopes. For a significant number of them, the ulcers were likely to return as soon as thalidomide treatment stopped, which many found they were forced to do because of the drug's side effects. After all, following four weeks of treatment with thalidomide, up to 50% of patients were already likely to be experiencing thalidomide-induced neuropathy. This was of considerable concern to Dr. Debra Birnkrant of the FDA, who wrote a critical report on the subject published in the *New England Journal of Medicine* in 1997.[401] She pointed in particular to the large number of 'major adverse events' associated with this treatment, which for two of the patients in one study included Grade 4 neutropenia. Neutropenia describes a reduction in the number of white blood cells, and of course this effect was compounded by the fact that at the same time thalidomide acted as a sedative on many patients. The problem here was this: sedating HIV/AIDS patients who already often have low energy levels is not a helpful treatment, and neither is reducing the white blood cell count of people suffering from a disease of the immune system. In fact, the whole concept of giving a medication believed to suppress the immune system to people suffering from immune-system disease is dubious in the extreme, akin to giving a nerve poison to people with a progressive nervous system disease as happened with leprosy. It will never be known how many HIV/AIDS patients were speeded to their deaths by thalidomide following the misguided enthusiasm for this product, nor how many ended their days in misery needlessly suffering the serious side effects of thalidomide, including polyneuritis and other complications.

Thalidomide, blood clots and heart attacks

In December 2012, a team of doctors treating an HIV-associated Aphthous ulcer patient made the discovery that thalidomide had caused dangerous deep vein thrombosis in a 48-year-old man. They felt they

[401] Birnkrant D. (1997), 'Thalidomide for Aphthous Ulcers in HIV Infection', *New England Journal of Medicine* 337: 1086-1087.

should warn others of this risk, which was new to them,[402] although well-known to anyone who had studied the wider effects of the drug. After all, already during the trial of Chemie Grünenthal executives in the late 1960s and early 1970s, it was reported that a Dr. Konrad Lang had used thalidomide on children with learning disabilities at the University Clinic in Bonn from early 1957 over a period of at least two years. The children were treated with up to 20 times the normal adult doses of thalidomide, and out of the core treatment group of 40 children, three died from heart or circulatory failure and one became blind for a time.[403] Dr. Lang considered this was not the fault of thalidomide. But it probably was, as evidence of such problems has in the meantime become undeniable. A 2009 report in the *Journal of Clinical Oncology,* for instance, said that myeloma patients taking thalidomide were at high risk of developing blood clots (as many as one in two), with obvious risks to life.[404] The risk of blood clotting caused by thalidomide, though, was already well-known: a 2002 study of 23 myeloma patients being treated with thalidomide found seven developed blood clots (thromboembolism).[405] In fact, when the incidence rate of thromboembolism observed in this study is compared against treatment time, the patients receiving thalidomide could have been 14 times as likely to get a venous or arterial thromboembolism as patients not receiving the drug.

Although these were very serious findings, however, they did not reveal the full extent of the problem. In April 2011, the Korean Food and Drug Administration published a warning that thalidomide could cause myocardial infarctions (heart attacks) and cerebrovascular disease (strokes).[406] This warning was also published in Germany: Celgene sent a letter to health professionals there advising them of these risks, and

[402] Hodowanec A.C., Han A., Barker D.E., Rubenstein P.G., Max B. (2012), 'Thalidomide-Associated Thrombosis in the Treatment of HIV-Associated Severe Aphthous Disease: A Case Report and Review of the Literature', *J. Int. Assoc. Phsyicians AIDS Care (Chic)* 2012 Nov-Dec; 11(6):345-7.

[403] Dagmar and Karl-Heinz Wenzel, *Der Contergan-Prozess;* testimony of Dr. Konrad Lang, volume II, pp. 122-127. Doses rates reported of 10-20 milligrams per kilogram of body weight. A child weighing 30 kg could have been dosed with 600 mg of thalidomide at these rates, or 24 normal Contergan tablets.

[404] Anna Flanga, Marina Marchetti (2009) 'Venous Thromboembolism in the Hematologic Malignancies', *Journal Clinical Oncology* vol 27 no. 29 4848-4857 (14 September 2009).

[405] Bowcock S.J., Rassam S.M., Ward S.M., Turner J.T., Laffan M. (2002) 'Thromboembolism in patients on thalidomide for myeloma', *Hematology,* 2002 Feb; 7 (1):51-3.

[406] 'Warning against thalidomide posted', *The Korea Herald* (28 April 2011).

recommending the use of anti-clotting agents.[407] The public warnings and advice came at least nine years after a credible and published piece of research highlighted this area of risk, but in reality, the risks were evident from at least the time of Dr. Lang's lethal research at the University Clinic in Bonn, which suggests the question: how could doctors using the drug in 2012 have been unaware of these risks?

But before we go on, we have to explore a third potential link between the ENL and the AIDS stories in relation to thalidomide. It centres on the person of Dr. Gilla Kaplan, a graduate of Hebrew University Jerusalem who had most probably (given that she was 67 years old in 2014) studied there at the time when Professor Sheshkin was carrying out his work with thalidomide.[408] This connection to Sheshkin is even more likely given the fact that Kaplan herself studied the use of thalidomide in treatment of leprosy patients, observing that it appeared to inhibit a substance named 'Tumour Necrosis Factor – alpha' (TNF-α), produced by white blood cells as part of the body's natural immune response to disease. If this was so, then it could assist in a wide range of diseases, including tuberculosis, arthritis and AIDS. As the story is told, it was Kaplan who informed the Celgene division of Celanese Corporation about this interesting set of potential effects and gave Celgene the idea of applying for a licence to make and distribute thalidomide in the USA,[409] which it did in 1998. She was appointed to the Celgene board in that same year and has retained this connection with the company ever since, although it was not long before it was discovered that thalidomide was also capable of causing an increase in TNF-α production, throwing this whole area into doubt.[410] Regardless, she flourished: in 2013 *Forbes* reported that her total compensation as a director of Celgene for that year was US $822,181.[411] We will examine the full implications of the Celgene connection shortly.

[407] Letter containing 'Wichtige Information für Angehörige der Heilberufe über das Auftreten von Thromboembolien im Zusammenhang mit Thalidomide Celgene. (Thalidomid)', issued by Celgene, Munchen, April 2011.

[408] *http://www.forbes.com/profile/gilla-kaplan* <viewed 10 November 2014>.

[409] Hawthorne F., *Inside the FDA: The Business and Politics Behind the Drugs We Take and the Food We Eat,* (NY: John Wiley, 2005), pp. 110-111.

[410] Shannon E, Noveck R, Sandoval F, Kamath B. (2008) 'Thalidomide suppressed IL-1beta while enhancing TNF-alpha and IL-10 when cells in whole blood were stimulated with lipopolysaccharide', *Immunopharmacol Immunotoxicol* 2008; 30(3):447-57.

[411] *http://www.forbes.com/profile/gilla-kaplan* <view 10 November 2014>.

Thalidomide and cancer

Beginning with research reported by Dr. Keller in August 1954, Grünenthal had been trying to establish anti-cancer properties for thalidomide and thalidomide-like drugs, and in the late 1990s this area of activity finally took off. The cancer in question was a rare blood disease, multiple myeloma. As with the deployment of thalidomide in leprosy therapy, there was a 'champion' for its use for treating myeloma: Bart Barlogie, a professor at the University of Arkansas, published a number of articles that produced favourable headlines about the benefits of thalidomide in myeloma therapy.[412]

In fact, an article published on 16 February 2010 in a web-based journal for multiple myeloma patients, *The Myeloma Beacon,* even reported that Barlogie had actually *cured* multiple myeloma using thalidomide. The claims were, however, overblown. Originally titled 'Multiple Myeloma Total Therapy Regime Claims 50 Percent Cure Rate', the piece drew complaints because this headline did not match the content, and it was therefore retitled 'Total Therapy Regime May Be Highly Effective in Newly Diagnosed Myeloma Patients'.[413] Even after the amendments, Barlogie was quoted as hoping he would find a cure for multiple myeloma, but there is no evidence to date that he has done so.

Indeed, his optimism and enthusiasm for thalidomide for treating this disease seem to have influenced his interpretation of his results, which, if we look at them critically, are in fact much less positive than at first glance. For example, in one of Barlogie's most prominent papers, published in the *New England Journal of Medicine* in March 2006, he reported that a follow-up of survivors at 42 months showed 'complete response' rates of 62% among the thalidomide-treated patients, whereas rates were just 43% among those not treated with thalidomide. That looks like a tremendous result in favour of thalidomide! But then the article goes on to note that among the patients who had relapses, thalidomide patients survived 1.1 years whereas non-thalidomide patients survived 2.7 years. So, in this circumstance, thalidomide patients died much quicker than those who had not taken the drug! The paper concludes with this statement:

412 See, e.g., Bart Barlogie et al. (2006) 'Thalidomide and Hematopoietic-Cell Transplantation for Multiple Myeloma', *NEJM* Vol 354:1021-1030 (9 March 2006).

413 *http://www.myelomabeacon.com/news/2010/02/16/multiple-myeloma-total-therapy-regimen-claims-50-percent-cure-rate* <viewed 7 January 2013>.

> *When incorporated into high-dose therapy for myeloma, thalidomide increased the frequency of complete responses and extended event-free survival at the expense of added adverse effects without improving overall survival.*[414]

Again, this sounds very positive, although the odd formulation 'event-free survival at the expense of added adverse effects' is an indication that there is some fine print here. In fact, the 'added adverse effects' include:

- thrombosis or embolism, affecting 30% of the thalidomide group and only 17% of the non-thalidomide group;
- bowel obstruction affecting 14% of the thalidomide group and 8% of the non-thalidomide group; and
- peripheral neuropathy affecting 27% of the thalidomide group and 17% of the non-thalidomide group.

What is more, after two years of treatment around half of the thalidomide patients had dropped out or died, and this increased to about two-thirds after three years.[415] This is important: after all, once patients 'drop out' of a study, usually because of adverse effects of treatment, what happens to them subsequently ceases to be recorded, and the final results are valid only for those who have stayed the full course. Thus, the '5-year survival' figures headlined in the media do not represent the underlying realities of the study, and the adverse effect rates listed above must therefore certainly understate the reality of what happens on thalidomide treatment.

Less well-publicised reports tell a completely different story about the merits of thalidomide in myeloma treatment. One high-quality report published in 2013 is a meta-analysis of randomised trials in relation to such treatment. Here the authors explain how they scrutinised 73 papers that compared the Melphalan-Prednisone and Thalidomide (MPT) treatment advocated by Barlogie and others with the version of that treatment that excluded thalidomide. They found, however, only seven that reported trials that were well enough designed and executed to provide a reliable basis for analysis and comparison. What is more, only six of those studies proved methodologically close enough to one another to enable this analysis. In other words, 90% of

[414] Bart Barlogie et al. (2006) 'Thalidomide and Hematopoietic-Cell Transplantation for Multiple Myeloma', *NEJM* Vol 354:1021-1030, March 9 2006.
[415] *Ibid.*

these 73 studies on the use of thalidomide in cancer treatment were considered *not* to be the result of reliable and robust science.[416]

But the analysis of the six usable reports was revealing. They covered a total of 1,685 patients in all, and on this basis, the researchers doing the meta-analysis calculated survival until date of death, or until the date the patient was last known to be alive. They found that neuropathy occurred at five times the rate in thalidomide patients (15% versus 3%), and deep vein thrombosis occurred at three times the rate (6% versus 2%). What is more, 35% of thalidomide patients gave up treatment because of adverse effects, while non-haematologic adverse events (i.e. infections etc.) happened to 40% of patients treated with thalidomide as against 18% of the others. Despite these findings, the authors concluded that patients on the thalidomide treatment had a 'better outcome' even while at the same time admitting that these patients were at risk of 'severe adverse events'.[417]

One wonders what the definition of 'better' is here, but we have to admit that the mainly elderly people who have myeloma are very sick, and that there are a number of diverse factors that can have an impact on their treatment and the progression of their disease. It is also true that the decision about whether to use thalidomide as part of a treatment for myeloma is certainly far from being clear cut and involves a serious consideration of quality of life issues compared to length of life, though from this evidence it appears that thalidomide is very likely to impair both.

Cui bono? Follow the money!

These cases of thalidomide being used enthusiastically to treat very different diseases and causing a range of 'adverse effects' share a common trajectory, and that is in fact very similar to the very first of the drug's 'killer apps' as a 'safe' sedative in the late 1950s and early 1960s. Initial overblown reports of thalidomide's therapeutic effectiveness that ignore the likelihood – and eventually the certainty – of its often devastating side effects lead to a large-scale consumption of the drug. Scientific reports then emerge confirming those side effects, leading eventually to the conclusion 'No Role for Thalidomide in

[416] Antonio Palumbo et al. (2013) 'Safety of thalidomide in newly diagnosed elderly myeloma patients: a meta-analysis of data from individual patients in six randomised trials', *Haematologica* 2013; 98(1) pp. 87-94.
[417] *Ibid.*

Leprosy'[418] in the case of ENL, although the drug's use in myeloma therapy continues.

Clearly, the misplaced enthusiasm had to come from somewhere, and although scientists and doctors have led the way in promoting adoption of thalidomide therapies, it was manufacturers of the drug who supplied those wanting to develop and make use of such therapies and who also had a keen and obvious interest in ensuring that the drug's use was as widespread as possible.

From late 1961 until the 1990s, the only company known to manufacture and supply thalidomide in commercial quantities was Chemie Grünenthal, which in 2003 claimed it had 'provid[ed] thalidomide free of charge' until its 'reserves' from 1961 had been 'exhausted, [and] we are no longer able to provide this aid'.[419] We have already seen that the statement's implication that manufacturing stopped in 1961 is certainly untrue, and that the claim that the company provided it without charge is extremely unlikely; indeed a newspaper report from 1972 indicated that the company was thinking in terms of renewed commercialisation of the drug.[420] There is, though, additional evidence to support the belief that while they may indeed have supplied the drug free to researchers, the company was in fact making money from sales of thalidomide until after 2000.

For one thing, Grünenthal's thalidomide development programme, as evidenced by the patents we have mentioned earlier, tracked developments in the USA in the 1980s and beyond, in relation to AIDS and cancer therapies, extremely closely. In fact, two of the Grünenthal scientists listed on the company's patents for anti-cancer applications for thalidomide-related compounds in the 1990s, Professor Kurt Eger and Dr. Uwe Teubert, went on to be listed on a series of American and Canadian patents covering certain anti-cancer properties of the drug that were filed between 2002 and 2007. (See Appendix 3.) Based on this evidence, it certainly does not appear as if Grünenthal has even now abandoned its commercial interest in this drug in spite of its grand pronouncement to the contrary in 2003.

418 Crawford, C.L. (1994) 'Use of Thalidomide in Leprosy', *Adverse Drug and Toxicological Reviews* 13(4):177-192; World Health Organisation, Leprosy Team, May 2003; 'No Role for Thalidomide in Leprosy', The Pan American Health Organisation: *http://www.paho.org/English/AD/DPC/CD/thalidomide.htm* <viewed 21 July 2011>.

419 In a letter from Grünenthal to Dr. Claes Malm, Haematology Clinic, Linköping, Sweden dated 2003-08-02 (copy of letter held by the Thalidomide Trust).

420 'Contergan-Firma bekämpft Lepra; Chemie Grünenthal verschenkt Thalidomide an bedürftige Länder', *Ruhr Nachrichten* (18 July 1972).

But there is also circumstantial evidence that the company benefitted from its longstanding Latin American connections in relation to the illicit market for thalidomide supplies in the USA during the 1990s. Grünenthal, after all, registered and maintained an extensive set of thalidomide trade names, with the most obvious trademarks for mono-preparations (drugs that only contain thalidomide such as Softenon), throughout the entire period. In Venezuela, Softenon was registered in 1958, Peracon in 1959 and Enterosediv in 1998. In Brazil, Enterosediv was registered in 1973 and Softenon in 1982. In Colombia, Softenon was registered in 1978, Softenil in 1980, Enterosediv in 1980 and Softenon re-registered in 1983. In Chile, the company registered Softenon in 1979 and Enterosediv in 1998. In Argentina, the firm registered Softenon in 1980 and Enterosediv in 1998.[421] Here, we have also identified a drug registration for a new thalidomide mono-preparation under the name Talidomida Cassara by Grünenthal Argentina withdrawn in 1999.[422] The company was therefore in a position to sell thalidomide under a bewildering variety of brand names throughout Latin America at exactly the time thalidomide smuggling into the USA for HIV/AIDS took off in the 1980s and 1990s.

There is still more evidence in support of this. In 2006, for instance, Grünenthal reported having seven subsidiary companies in Latin America, mostly established during the 1990s, again when the AIDS thalidomide black market in the USA was at its peak. These subsidiaries are located in Argentina, Mexico, Peru, Chile, Colombia, Venezuela and Ecuador.[423] The company's ties with Ecuador are particularly strong: they have had a subsidiary there since 1972, and in 2007 Michael Wirtz, the honorary consul for Ecuador in North Rhine Westphalia and the family head of Grünenthal, was honoured with the Ecuadorian National Order of Merit in recognition of his philanthropic

[421] The various national trademark registration details may be found in Appendix 4.

[422] The database of the Argentinean drug authority, ANMAT, consulted on 11 December 2011 *(http://www.anmat.gov.ar/aplicaciones_net/applications/consultas/consultas/consulta_puntual.htm)* shows three thalidomide mono-preparations under the product name Talidomida Cassara. The manufacturer is stipulated as Grünenthal Argentina S.A. The records do not show when the licence commenced, only that it was withdrawn in December 1999 and still active until August 2002. However, the product number shows a low (and therefore early) serial, 2,966. This shows that it had been registered for possibly some decades, as the most recent thalidomide product – from a different manufacturer - had the much higher serial 39,680. The conditions of sale for the Grünenthal product also indicate an early registration, as it was to be provided 'under archived prescription', whereas most of the other providers of thalidomide had the additional condition 'exclusive use in hospitals'.

[423] *Der Eigene Weg*, Grünenthal 60th Anniversary publication (2006), p. 13.

work in the country. In 2005, the company opened a new production plant in Ecuador, intended to be the hub for all company activities in Latin America, at a cost of US $7.5 million.[424]

However, the firm that has benefitted most financially from the thalidomide booms of the late 1990s to the present was not Grünenthal, but an American company named Celgene. The background to this is highly significant and suggestive, if a bit convoluted. US-based Celanese Corporation, which mainly manufactured industrial chemicals, was taken over by Hoechst, a former part of IG Farben, in 1986. Celanese's Celgene division, which had hitherto focused on environmental biotechnology such as enzymes used to clear up pollutants, was then separated from its parent, becoming an independent publicly listed company through an IPO in 1987. In the years that followed, Hoechst, the company behind all this, itself engaged in a series of organisational changes, eventually merging with Rhône-Poulenc of France in 1999 to form Aventis Deutschland (which later became Sanofi Aventis). Just before that merger, in 1998, the same year in which Dr. (now Professor) Gilla Kaplan became a director of Celgene, the FDA awarded Celgene a licence to market thalidomide for use with ENL in the USA. In 2008, Celgene acquired Pharmion of UK, the company which held the EU licence for thalidomide, thus becoming the world's leading producer of thalidomide and its derivatives. By this time, Chemie Grünenthal was completely out of the picture as far as thalidomide was concerned (although its employees were still registering some patents). We do not know why all of this played out the way it did, but we will consider some possibilities in the conclusion to this chapter.

In the meantime, though, it is worth pausing in the narrative briefly to consider three key facts, and a question that arises from these facts. The first is that thalidomide finally got FDA approval for use in the United States in 1998 after having failed to do so when Richardson Merrell applied for it in the early 1960s. The second fact is that the FDA approval in the United States was for treatment of ENL, a complication of leprosy, a disease that is extremely rare in that country. The third key fact is that thalidomide has become a very profitable product for Celgene, *which seems odd considering that it received FDA approval only for treatment of a rare disease.* Indeed, sales by the firm amounted to a whopping US $36 million plus per month in the third

[424] Grünenthal press releases, 2007, 2005.

quarter of 2013,[425] and in 2015 sales of Celgene's thalidomide-based medicines amounted to an estimated US $6.97 billion, over three-quarters of the firm's total sales that year.[426]

Here is the question that emerges when we take all of these facts into consideration: *How did all of this happen?* The answer is fairly straightforward: impressive financial results were achieved for the most part though 'off label' sales involving the unlicensed treatment of a large variety of cancers. The FDA issued a stern warning to Celgene about this in 2000 and also expressed concerns (yet again) at the time about thalidomide neuropathy.[427] The firm appears to have either overcome or ignored these objections by 2008, when it announced at a public meeting that the drug was being used for treatment of 25 cancers,[428] despite the fact that by then, only one cancer type – multiple myeloma – had been licensed for treatment by the FDA. Indeed, overall off-label sales have accounted for 95% of total sales of thalidomide between 1998 and 2007.[429] A whistle-blower's allegations about the moves by the company to promote off-label use of thalidomide-based medicines, which may well have been illegal, are being investigated in a US court.[430]

But there was another reason that sales volumes became so healthy for the firm: astonishing price increases. A blog post written in April 2010 by a myeloma sufferer called 'Lance' living in Canada, for instance, pointed out that thalidomide was being sold at CA $400 for a

425 'Celgene Reports Record Third Quarter 2009 Operating and Financial Results', *Reuters,* 22 October 2009: http://uk.reuters.com/article/celgene-idUKN2150586120091022 <viewed 8 January 2013>.

426 Jef Feeley and Doni Bloomfield, 'Court to hear whistleblower's case alleging Celgene's aggressive push of Thalidomide,' Chigago Tribune (22 August 2016), available at: *http://www.chicagotribune.com/news/sns-wp-blm-thalidomide-6320256a-6888-11e6-91cb-ecb5418830e9-20160822-story.html* <viewed 19 September 2016>.

427 Warning letter issued to John W. Jackson CEO of Celgene on 2 April 2000 from Thomas W. Abrams, Director, Division of Drug Marketing, Advertising and Communications, Food and Drug Administration, Rockville MD. Available at: *http://www.fda.gov/downloads/Drugs/GuidanceComplianceRegulatoryInformation/EnforcementActivitiesbyFDA/WarningLettersandNoticeofViolationLetterstoPharmaceuticalCompanies/UCM165843.pdf* <viewed 10 February 2016>.

428 Presentation by Dr. Sol. J. Barer, CEO of Celgene to conference of the Thalidomide Victims' Association of Canada, 7 November 2008.

429 Meeting Report Celgene – Revlimid; Institute of Directors (London) 26 January 2007 Present: Mr. Simon Vane-Percy (Vane Percy & Roberts (Communication Consultants)); Dr. David Stirling (Celgene) Dr. Claus Newman & Dr. Martin Johnson (Thalidomide Trust) figure of 99.5% sales for Multiple Myeloma quoted, for which at that time a license was not held.

430 Jef Feeley and Doni Bloomfield, 'Court to hear whistleblower's case alleging Celgene's aggressive push of Thalidomide', *Chigago Tribune* (22 August 2016), available at: *http://www.chicagotribune.com/news/sns-wp-blm-thalidomide-6320256a-6888-11e6-91cb-ecb5418830e9-20160822-story.html* <viewed 19 September 2016>.

month's supply in 1999, CA $800 in 2002, CA $1,500 in 2003, CA $3,600 in 2005 and CA $4,000 in 2010, a tenfold increase in just eleven years. By then, the Canadian healthcare system had long since refused to pay for the treatment. Lance went on to note that a fellow myeloma sufferer with whom he was in contact had traced a supplier in Mexico who offered thalidomide for US $90 per month, but Lance was blocked from importing the drug into Canada.[431] The situation was similar in the United States, where a month's treatment cost more than US $3,000 in 2008. The company justified these massive costs (and cost increases) by pointing to the requirement of having a strict patient protection programme in place (STEPS), which added considerably to the price of the product, although the fact that the firm itself had insisted that this programme be put in place was not highlighted quite so prominently. Clearly, though, Celgene's approach to marketing the drug differed fundamentally not only from the early Grünenthal one, but also from the low-cost strategy deployed in Brazil and elsewhere in the Third World. But the importance of these off-label sales for Celgene's overall income stream from thalidomide also underscores the fact that yet again the drug has been involved in what is essentially a large-scale experiment with human subjects.

The never-ending experiment

The prominence of off-label sales of thalidomide is all the more remarkable because of this stunning fact: to the present day, no one knows how the drug actually works or why it causes the problems that it does. This was stated most baldly on 7 November 2008 when Dr. Sol J. Barer, the then CEO and Chairman of Celgene, addressed a conference of the Thalidomide Victims' Association of Canada (TVAC). Among other things, he made the point that the drug was currently being used to treat some 25 different types of cancer in the United States. In answer to a question from the floor, though, Barer replied that the molecular action of the drug in the human body was still unknown.[432] This was astonishing, given the lengthy history of the drug and the variety of uses it has been put to, but this position has been

[431] *http://thecancerdiariesmm.blogspot.co.uk/2010/04/shame-on-you.html* <viewed 7 January 2013>.

[432] Presentation by Dr. Sol. J. Barer, CEO of Celgene to conference of the Thalidomide Victims' Association of Canada, 7 November 2008. The question was posed by Martin Johnson, co-author of this book.

reiterated consistently in various independent research papers. For instance:

> *...its [thalidomide's] exact mode of action, however, is not known...*[433]

> *...while thalidomide's mechanism of action still remains unknown...*[434]

There is, however, no question that some of the side effects of taking the drug are all too well known, and that most of them have been known for a very long time. From the first reports of adverse side effects, it was clear that thalidomide acted on the peripheral nervous system causing polyneuritis, and the common side effect of severe constipation could indicate a pronounced effect on the parasympathetic nervous system. This pattern of side effects, otherwise known as thalidomide neuropathy, must by now have affected millions of adults.

Of course, the most famous effect is the range of birth defects caused by the drug when it is taken by pregnant women. Over the years, researchers have proposed various theories of how the drug acted to cause this damage. In 2011, the *American Registry of Pathology* published a review of these theories about how thalidomide causes malformations in the foetus and concluded that the most feasible mechanism is that it damages key nerve cells in the embryonic neural crest which then prevent the subsequent development of the associated limbs and organs.[435] This theory had been developed initially by Professor Janet McCredie (Sydney) in conjunction with Professor Hans Willert (Göttingen), who built on an original observation that the 'missing' bone structure in thalidomide children corresponded closely with the areas of segmental nerve supply of the skeleton. They then theorised that thalidomide caused the damage to the unborn children by acting as a nerve poison (neurotoxin) on the neural crest of the developing foetus.[436] The neural crest is a structure within the embryo which develops along the length of the spinal cord, forming the

433 O. Rick, T. Braun, W Siegert, J. Beyer (2006) 'Activity of thalidomide in patients with platinum-refractory germ-cell tumours', *European Journal of Cancer* 42(2006) 1775-1779.

434 N.A. Thadani, J.P. McNamee, L.M. Winn (2006) 'Thalidomide alters c-MYB and PIM-1 signaling in K-562 cells', *Pharmacological Research* 54 (2006) 91-96.

435 Michael J. Klein, S. Fiona Bonar, Tony Freemont, Tuyethoa N. Vinh, Robert Lopez-Ben, Herrick J. Siegel, Gene P. Siegal (2011) 'Non-Neoplastic Diseases of Bones and Joints', *Atlas of NonTumor Pathology*, First Series Fascicle 9 pp. 171-181 American Registry of Pathology in association with the Armed Forces Institute of Pathology, Washington DC.

436 McCredie, J., *Beyond Thalidomide; birth defects explained.* (London: RSM, 2007).

autonomic and peripheral nervous systems,[437] so there is a logical connection between this structure and effects such as polyneuritis and the other well-known thalidomide effects linked with the parasympathetic nervous system, including the digestive tract and the circulatory system.

However, in spite of this review of the literature and science, the jury is still out on the precise mechanism by which the drug causes birth defects. An expert conference convened by the WHO on Thalidomide Embryopathy in Geneva in February 2014 reviewed the neural crest and other main theories that have been propounded and concluded that the available evidence on the mechanism of action of thalidomide in fact does not support the neural crest theory. The conference, which drew together the majority of the world's published scientific experts on the recognition of thalidomide damage and the mechanisms by which it has been found to operate on babies in the womb, concluded that the precise mechanism by which this occurs remains unknown but is probably connected with the way in which it bonds with a protein named Cereblon, which is involved in cell growth and development.[438]

In other words, Celgene's CEO, Dr. Barer, was right when he said in 2008 that the drug's mechanism of action remained unknown, even in relation to the way it causes birth defects, which makes the global sales and marketing efforts undertaken with regard to this drug even more extraordinary. Having discussed the situation in Brazil, those attending the 2014 WHO conference considered the current manufacture of the drug in countries such as Indonesia and India, and the possibility that a lack of birth defect reporting in such countries meant that thalidomide birth defect epidemics could already be taking place there. Among the conclusions they reached was this:

> *Increasing availability of thalidomide, particularly its use in countries with limited drug regulation (because of its important use in leprosy treatment), is the cause of a new wave of fetal*

[437] 'The term *neural crest* refers to an embryologic structure that develops from cells that originate from the thin lateral margins of the neural plate. These cells migrate to the midline dorsal to the neural tube to form the neural crest and then continue to migrate in the body to give rise to the primary sensory neurons of the dorsal root ganglia of the spinal nerves (Carpenter-1983).' See *http://braininfo.rprc.washington.edu/centraldirectory.aspx?ID=1366* <viewed 16 June 2017>.

[438] *http://www.who.int/medicines/news/thalidomide_embryopathy_meeting_report.pdf?ua=1* <viewed 10 November 2014>.

malformations, either during a clinically indicated use or by accidental/off-label use by unintended users.[439]

Conclusions

Almost immediately after the thalidomide disaster came to light with a vengeance in November 1961, Grünenthal scientists led by their chief, Heinrich Mückter, began work on developing the drug further, exploring a very wide range of possible uses. During the forty years that followed, Grünenthal was at the forefront of exploring practically every new potential application of thalidomide that has ultimately become newsworthy, from leprosy to cancer treatments. From the late 1960s through the 1980s, the company was furthermore undoubtedly manufacturing and supplying the drug worldwide, and encouraging researchers – particularly in Third World countries – to test the drug out on some particularly vulnerable patients.

By the 1990s, at the height of the HIV/AIDS crisis, Grünenthal's already existing Latin American subsidiaries along with new ones established during that decade were thriving, and a considerable amount of the thalidomide they produced was being smuggled into the USA, with an impact on yet another group of vulnerable patients. We are not saying necessarily that the thalidomide used in this way came directly from Grünenthal's subsidiaries – we cannot prove this – but we can say with certainty that the initial availability of the drug in Latin America was a result of Grünenthal's work over the previous few decades, and that furthermore there was as yet no other company producing the drug in commercial quantities. It is clear, then, that regardless of their responsibility for those damaged by thalidomide in AIDS therapy, the company and its staff must shoulder the primary responsibility for the second phase of the thalidomide birth defect catastrophe in Brazil, and probably, too, for any additional epidemics yet to be discovered elsewhere in the world.

But the company is now joined by another culprit. Celgene's success in gaining FDA approval for use of the drug to combat ENL in the United States in 1998 was followed a few years later by Chemie Grünenthal's withdrawal from the thalidomide market. By 2008, through acquisition of a British firm with the EU rights to the drug, Celgene was the leading producer of thalidomide worldwide, profiting

[439] *Ibid.*

enormously, primarily from non-approved, 'off-label' usage of thalidomide for cancer treatments.

Celgene continues to operate in a macabre, extraordinarily unfortunate but also consistent pattern that has characterised the drug's history. Thalidomide is first hailed as a wonder therapy for treatment of some new disease until gradually the problems of the side effects emerge yet again, and the drug moves on to yet another new disease. And *plus ça change, plus c'est la même chose:* regardless of the new disease targeted, the side effects do not change, and they include peripheral neuropathy, heart and circulatory problems, bowel obstructions and – still in the 21st century – birth defects.

We do not know why and how Celgene displaced Chemie Grünenthal in this area during the late 1990s and the first decade of the 21st century. But it is intriguing to think that this, too, might be a case of *plus ça change, plus c'est la même chose.* After all, Celgene is a company that was founded after the takeover of its parent company, Celanese, by former IG Farben member Hoechst. The German company then merged with French Rhône-Poulenc to form Sanofi Aventis, although the two shared connections with one another from much earlier, extending back to joint participation in medical experimentation on concentration camp inmates during the Second World War. And now Celgene, affiliated with Sanofi Aventis, is making billions of dollars through sales of thalidomide, functioning in effect as the true heir to the Contergan story that began at the latest with Rhône-Poulenc's licensing of that trade name to Chemie Grünenthal.

Figure 14: Mat Fraser, aged 6.
Mat went on to become a professional actor and musician.

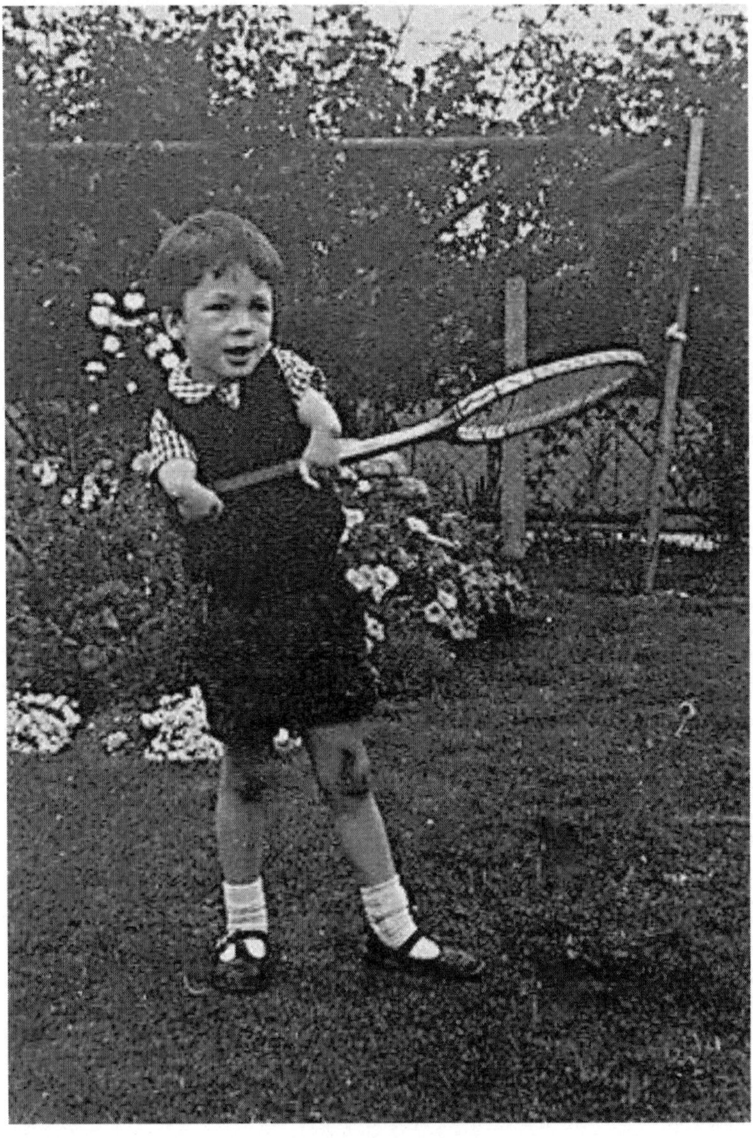

© M Fraser

Conclusion

WE BEGAN THIS BOOK WITH AN ACCOUNT of just how dreadful the thalidomide catastrophe really was. It constituted a global disaster on a scale that has never been considered in its full dimensions before, with upwards of 150,000 babies estimated to have been destroyed or injured. Some 25,000 of them were born alive, but most died as babies or during childhood. We reviewed the level of nerve injuries to adults, noting that the numbers so affected must have been in the hundreds of thousands.

We then saw how, as the catastrophe unfolded in each country where thalidomide was commercialised, it was treated as a local problem, usually for the licensee companies and the national governments to deal with on a piecemeal basis. We observed how the original marketing and distribution of the drug using many different companies and scores of different brand names served to confuse the public, and how these different names and delays in informing the public in some countries contributed to babies being born affected by the drug long after the terrible effects it caused had been made known, while simultaneously making it harder for many to seek redress for their loss and injury.

We saw that for most families affected – those whose babies had miscarried, been stillborn (even possibly killed in the hospitals) or survived birth, but not lived long enough to be recognised by the various national settlement schemes – there was no justice, no compensation. Delays of over ten years in most jurisdictions in arriving at the original settlements often caused very severe hardship and difficulties for the children and their families. The typical family in Germany, the UK and most other countries had to cope with caring for a thalidomide-injured child while confronting the challenges of their legal systems without anything more than the basic support for disabled children that their country might provide.

There is no question that these people were let down by their own legal systems which blocked speedy access to justice; by their governments which permitted the distribution of the drug; by the companies that licensed it and distributed it; and by the doctors and pharmacists who had supplied it. None of this was necessarily criminal, but it all served to protect the perpetrators of the crime, who have since gone to their graves unpunished. In the aftermath of the thalidomide disaster and to the present day, justice has not been delivered by national justice systems except in the most meagre way. Instead, what justice has been meted out has invariably come as a result of trial in the 'Court of Public Opinion'; only sustained media pressure and skilled political lobbying have thus far worked to secure some measure of justice – for those who have lived long enough to see it.

The results achieved through media and political pressure have themselves all been based on clear presentations of the evidence available, evidence which the representatives of Grünenthal in their public statements have sought to deny even in the most recent times. Contrary to what the company continues to maintain, however, when the decision was made to produce thalidomide, there *was* widespread knowledge about the effects of analogous drugs, and the potential side-effects should therefore have been predictable. We have demonstrated that in fact these effects were not only predicted, but widely predicted, and not only by Dr. Frances Kelsey of the US Food and Drug Administration, but by many others, including Professor Aygun of Turkey, East German scientific authorities, Professor Riemschneider with his animal experiments and even advisers to Grünenthal themselves. Indeed, the research commissioned by the Distillers Company, the UK licensee for thalidomide, which was published in the *Lancet* in January 1958, also made the risks associated with the drug plain.

Grünenthal has been steadfast in its claim that it tested the drug according to the standards of the time. The firm's representatives have also indicated that such testing was minimal and performed only on animals, but, as we have shown, descriptions of the drug in patents strongly suggest otherwise. We have demonstrated that in many of the earliest patents filed by Grünenthal for thalidomide products there was a variety of descriptions of the potentially adverse effects of their drugs on the human nervous system. This information betrays the fact that the scientists concerned must have had access to human testing of these or very similar compounds. From their own evidence, as published in their patents, Grünenthal's scientists must have expected the drug to produce effects on the nervous systems of people taking thalidomide before they even released it into the market.

Unsurprisingly, virtually as soon as the drug started being tested and then widely sold in Germany and elsewhere, the company started to receive reports of nerve damage. Many credible reports of such injuries as a result of the use of the drug were available by 1959 at the latest, yet no moves were made to warn physicians or users about this side effect. We have seen how time and again the company resorted to outright denials that it had received any such reports. Nor was there any attempt to correct the erroneous notion that thalidomide was an effective sedative in relation to morning sickness experienced by pregnant women. As we have also seen, there is evidence that suspicions about the drug's role in causing birth defects were also articulated at an early juncture. Indeed, by 1959 at the latest, the company had received reports of thalidomide-related birth defects from a Dr. Kreideweiß, who contacted the company directly with his suspicions. Earlier still, there were danger signs, as highlighted in the test reports of Smith Kline & French in the United States in 1958 (see Chapter 1) and, even earlier, a thalidomide-damaged baby born to the wife of one of the company's own staff in December 1956. These reports and events were all ignored and also denied. The cover-up of the thalidomide catastrophe, in other words, started even as it began!

And this included government-level collusion. Suspicions about German government involvement in the manipulation of the trial of the Grünenthal executives and its strange ending have been in the public domain for over forty years, courtesy of *Thalidomide and the power of the drug companies* (1972) by Henning Sjöström and Robert Nilsson. These were no 'amateur' investigators, but instead active participants in the legal team working to represent Swedish thalidomide children and their families in the trial of the Astra company in Stockholm, which, as was detailed earlier in the book, had been brought to a successful and (relatively) early conclusion. Sjöström and Nilsson suggested, however, that one of the reasons the trial of Chemie Grünenthal executives lasted so long and was eventually suspended was the neglect of, and indifference to, the situation of thalidomiders on the part of West German government. In contrast, we have shown on the basis of newly discovered archival evidence that in fact there was active engagement with the trial on the part of the German federal government and the government of North Rhine Westphalia (NRW).

The documentary evidence that we have uncovered demonstrates clearly that leading members and departments of the West German government, in close cooperation with the NRW Justice Ministry, worked with Grünenthal and its attorneys – but not with the families affected by the thalidomide catastrophe – to establish the legal, regulatory and financial framework and resources for an eventual (and paltry) settlement offer, knowing that it represented at best 10% of the legitimate claims being made. Moreover, these powerful men and organisations worked together to engineer the suspension of the trial itself, in the face of official advice that such an action was almost certainly unlawful, indeed unconstitutional. And we have demonstrated that the settlement and the trial's suspension were inextricably related to one another in spite of the fact that the settlement of a *criminal* trial was at that time impossible under German Law.

We have shown unambiguously that there were clear instances of irregularities in relation to the conduct of the trial, and even likely corruption, especially on the part of authorities of the state of North Rhine Westphalia. Corruption, we freely admit, may seem an extreme charge, but evidence in regard to the role and conduct of Josef Neuberger is such that it is credible. Neuberger was the defence lawyer for Hermann Wirtz, eventually the leading defendant in the trial, when the indictment was being prepared in late 1966. Neuberger then became NRW Justice Minister and thus had ultimate responsibility for the prosecution of the trial. He gave up his position as defence attorney officially, but he did so without relinquishing his role in his law firm, which continued to defend Wirtz. And his State Secretary in the NRW Justice Ministry, Baron von Münchhausen, acted as a crucial conduit for information and decision-making in relation to the trial, the negotiation of a settlement and the trial's suspension, linking the Ministry, the prosecution, the federal government and the firm.

In what we can now see as a travesty of justice, the trial of Chemie Grünenthal executives in the late 1960s ended in December 1970 without a verdict. Despite this, the judges' report was damning about the company's actions in several respects, not least in confirming that those in charge of the company knew in 1959 at the latest that the drug had deleterious effects on users in terms of nerve damage. Specific points made by the judges in their report included the following:

- The company's testing of the drug was very inadequate by the standards of the day.

- Declaring the drug as 'completely non-toxic, atoxic and harmless' was negligent and not justified by previous testing.
- Chemie Grünenthal's top managers were guilty of negligent conduct, by failing to warn physicians against the potential nerve-damaging properties of thalidomide.

All in all, the court considered the overall conduct of the company negligent, and indicated that a drug manufacturer should be held responsible not only for pre-launch testing, but also for following up all aspects of the subsequent use of a drug. The judges were very explicit in this damning verdict:

> *The overall behaviour publicly shown by the company, Chemie Grünenthal, did not correspond with the standards required of a serious and conscientious producer of pharmaceuticals ... In the matter of nerve damage deviations from what is prescribed by law and justice were considerable ... The nerve damage would have been easy to foresee.*[440]

So, even though the court allowed the testimony of supposedly independent expert witnesses who in fact had close relationships with the accused while disallowing the testimony of Dr. Widekund Lenz, an independent expert who was one of those who made the link between thalidomide and birth defects, and even though defence attorneys and the company got away with attempts to intimidate journalists and witnesses, the judges put this damning opinion in writing in their justification for why they allowed the trial to be suspended. In other words, Grünenthal's public attempts to exonerate the firm's conduct were deemed false in a formal judicial opinion as long ago as 1971.

As we have shown, it is significant that the trial also cost an enormous amount of money, and furthermore that the firm agreed to pay all costs associated with it, something extremely unusual when a trial is suspended; state authorities almost invariably pay in such cases. Together with the relatively meagre (but, for the company, still expensive) compensation fund that Chemie Grünenthal and the German federal government put together for victims of thalidomide, these

[440] Quoted from the judgment by Henning Sjöström, Robert Nilsson, *Thalidomide and the power of the drug companies,* p. 265. The full judgment outlining the judges' opinions in relation to the suspension of the trial are in Medizinisch Pharmazeutische Studiengesellschaft e.V., Dokumentation III/71, 'Schriftlicher Einstellungsbeschluß der Ersten Großen Strafkammer des Landgerichts Aachen im sog. Contergan-Verfahren', Frankfurt, 1971, especially pp. 34-64.

expenditures – which have been estimated to have amounted in total to the equivalent of €300 million, six times the DM 100 million offered by the company to survivors[441] – exceeded the total value of the firm at the time. How this was financed remains a mystery. There are indications of approaches to other firms in the chemical and pharmaceutical industry for financial contributions to the settlement, undertaken by officials of the German federal government, but no evidence that these in fact were made. So, understanding just how Chemie Grünenthal survived this massive financial hit is a difficult task.

Here, the involvement of Otto Ambros (convicted as a war criminal at the Nuremberg IG Farben trial) in the company – latterly as a member of the supervisory board from 1976, in other words long after the withdrawal of thalidomide from most markets – may be relevant, not least because there are telling indications about his involvement in the catastrophe itself. For one thing, we have eyewitness testimony about his activities in the company several years prior to 1976. Moreover, his connection with Grünenthal's chairman, Hermann Wirtz, dated from 1960 at the latest, when they were both directors of another German drug company, Knoll AG. We have also seen, from Ambros's own written admission, that he was furthermore at some point a consultant to the Distillers Company, the British licensee for thalidomide. The Distillers Company was involved in the biochemical/pharmaceutical industry for only a short period starting around the time of the thalidomide catastrophe and withdrew completely from the area in its immediate aftermath. We can therefore reasonably surmise that Ambros was involved somehow in the whole process of managing first the marketing and licensing agreements that led to the spectacular commercial success of thalidomide, and then the damage limitation as it was withdrawn from sale.

Suspicions raised as a result of the details of the effects of thalidomide on humans in early patents of the drug, the involvement of Otto Ambros in Grünenthal, and specifically his responsibility for the introduction of nerve gas during the National Socialist period, led to our investigation of the 'prehistory' of thalidomide. Analysis of large numbers of patents for chemicals similar to thalidomide showed that many of them, all acting on the nervous system, were developed during

[441] Gregor Taxacher, 'Erfolgsstory mit katastrophalem Makel', WDR1 Themen, 23 November 2006, available at: *https://www1.wdr.de/archiv/contergan/contergan166.html* <viewed 7 March 2018>.

the Nazi period, some of which were related to nerve gas agent development, including the Rhône-Poulenc Antergan. Evidence submitted to the Astra trial in Sweden confirmed the fact that Contergan, similar in name and meaning to Antergan, was used by Grünenthal under agreement with Rhône-Poulenc.

We have, moreover, shown that the Wirtz brothers who founded Grünenthal, and their first chief scientist, Heinrich Mückter, formed an integral part of commercial, scientific and political networks active in Germany and German-occupied Europe in the Second World War. Here, they, along with many of those involved in pharmaceutical development in Nazi-dominated Europe, demonstrated levels of ruthlessness and brutality that would subsequently characterise the later introduction, sale and resistance to withdrawal of thalidomide, this in the face of mounting evidence of the harm it was doing, followed by a refusal to take responsibility when it finally was withdrawn. The conduct of the company towards its victims bore chilling comparison with the activities of Mückter and his colleagues in their work on typhus vaccine research in Poland. What is more, we saw that thalidomide was certainly not the first harmful drug Grünenthal had marketed. Indeed, one of the firm's first commercial successes was an extremely problematic antibiotic, which it refused to withdraw from sale even after alarms were raised about its effectiveness and side effects.

Although Mückter is seen by many as the central figure in the thalidomide story, we have demonstrated that in fact Professor Werner Schulemann of Bonn University played a pivotal role in it. He was at the centre of the scientific and commercial networks described above and carried out much work on thalidomide analogues. He trained Mückter and was instrumental in convincing the Wirtz family to set up Chemie Grünenthal in 1946 with Mückter as their chief scientist. He retained a close relationship with the company in the years that followed, appearing as an inventor on some of its patents. He also trained the young Herbert Keller, who joined Chemie Grünenthal from Bonn University in February 1954 and who, with Willi Kunz, appears as the co-inventor of thalidomide on the patent filed in Germany in May of that same year. As a supposedly independent expert, Schulemann also gave evidence at the trial.

Perhaps the most unexpected finding of all in our research, though, involved the uncovering of evidence surrounding Grünenthal's continuing role after 1961 in the development and production of thalidomide. It was astonishing to discover that the company's experience of the thalidomide catastrophe of the late 1950s and early 1960s did not stop the firm from continuing to market, distribute and develop the drug, seeking new uses for it into the 21st century. The concluding mystery here, for which we have not yet found an answer, is how the company benefited from this forty-year long programme of work, which led directly to the second generation thalidomide disaster, mainly focussing on Brazil.

So, where does this all leave us?

We should re-emphasise first of all that the evidence gathered in the course of research for this book and presented here was conducted largely in parallel with the great surge in campaigning on the part of the thalidomide survivors from 2007 onwards. We have described some of the many discouraging experiences they suffered over the years in trying to achieve justice, and how they finally devised effective strategies for presenting their story to the public and many different national governments, often with impressive results.

Here, we should note that thalidomide campaigners are not only concerned about compensation for the survivors that will help them manage the remainder of their lives, although this is clearly very important; they are also passionate about achieving some justice for all those thalidomide children 'who never made it', as well as for the parents and families who were affected. After all, the vast majority of families who had babies damaged by thalidomide have never been recognised or compensated in any way because the great majority of these children died before any of the settlement schemes took effect. And the settlement schemes were only concerned with those who had survived the many years until they actually began.

This is one way in which the research for and findings of this book have reinforced the work of campaigners, as illustrated perhaps most clearly in one conversation held early in the post-2000 campaigns where thalidomide representatives from a number of countries were present. One of the central discussion points involved the relevance of the Nazi connections of Grünenthal to what had happened. After all, as one participant pointed out, many German companies were active under the Nazi regime, such as Mercedes and BMW, observing that no one now thinks this past is relevant to how they operate today. After some deliberation, one of the Swedish thalidomiders countered with this statement: 'If Mercedes had built a car which killed ten thousand children they would not be around today.'[442] That summed up the feelings of those present, and the findings here suggest that Chemie Grünenthal should not be around today – and that it is a major injustice that it is.

Let us state this clearly one last time: the Nazi connections that led to the formation of Chemie Grünenthal and to the unfolding of the thalidomide catastrophe are both important and highly disturbing. Yet this is not the whole, nor even the most significant, aspect of the catastrophe. It was instead the astonishing discovery in 2014 of archival documents demonstrating that justice against Chemie Grünenthal and its managers was actively obstructed by the German federal and state governments whose responsibility it was to ensure that justice was done. The unavoidable conclusion is this: not only should Chemie Grünenthal finally be held to account for its role in the thalidomide disaster, so too should those authorities who failed to provide justice. Indeed, securing the latter may well enable the former.

One way forward towards resolving this would be if the German federal government were to establish a judicial review, which should be required to examine all the evidence available in the relevant archives, including material presented to the court in the trial, and also that which was gathered by the prosecution but not presented. Such a review could also consider additional evidence relevant to the case, such as has been uncovered in recent years in the archives of the German federal government and in those of the state of North Rhine Westphalia as well as documents gathered through discovery in a class-action suit on behalf of thalidomide survivors in Australia. On the basis of this review, we would expect confirmation of the general findings we have presented here (as well as some elaboration and refinement as well) in relation to the following questions:

- Did the company receive credible warnings from reputable sources about possible harm to people taking products containing thalidomide prior to main market launches in Germany (1 October 1957), UK (April 1958) and the other main

[442] The comment was made by Bjorn Håkansson to a German delegate at a discussion following the meeting in the Churchill Hotel London 30 January 2008 at which Martin Johnson was present. This was confirmed in conversation between Håkansson and Martin Johnson in October 2015.

countries concerned? And, if so, could they have anticipated the nature of the possible harm and its likely consequences?

- Just how many babies really were born damaged by thalidomide worldwide, and how many pregnancies overall were likely to have been affected?
- How many adults were harmed by thalidomide in all the countries where products containing thalidomide were distributed, and what are the consequences likely to have been for those people?
- Is it possible at this late time to take action against Grünenthal for its central role in what happened? Just what legal remedies are available to the German federal government in respect of the crimes committed by the company in the sale and distribution of products containing thalidomide?

All those connected with the consequences of this most terrible disaster can only hope that such a process will finally bring the truth about the thalidomide catastrophe properly into the open, and that justice will at last be done.

Figure 15: Philippa, showing the formidable independent spirit typical of many thalidomide survivors.

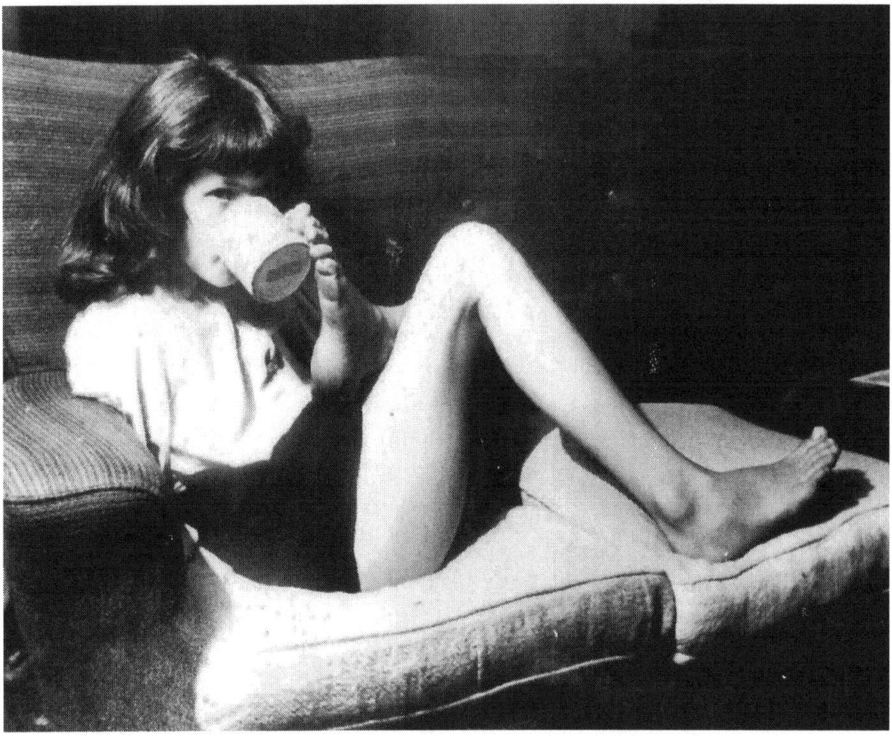

© News International (by kind permission); by agreement P. Verry

Appendix 1

Grünenthal thalidomide patents 1954-1960

Country	No.	Date of application	Title	Notes
West Germany	1074584	17 May 1954	Verfahren zur Herstellung von Derivaten von Amino-piperidin-2,6-dionen	Keller, Kunz
UK	768821	29 Apr 1955	Novel products of the Amino-piperidine-2,6-Dione Series	Inventor not named Ref Ge 1074584
Switzerland	336826	6 May 1955	Verfahren zur Herstellung von Derivaten von Amino-piperidin-2,6-dionen	Keller, Kunz Ref Ge 1074584
USA	2830991	16 May 1955	Products of the Amino-Piperidine-2,6-Dione Series	Keller, Kunz Ref Ge 1074584
France	1164512	17 May 1955	Procédé d'obtention de nouveaux produits de la série des amino-pipéridine-2,6-diones	Inventors not named Ref Ge 1074584
Sweden	190310	30 Jan 1956	Sätt att framställa farmakologiskt värdefulla piperidine-2,6-dioner	Keller, Kunz
Austria	193880	31 Jan 1956	Verfahren zur Herstellung von neuen Amino-piperidin-2,6-dionen	Keller, Kunz
Finland	15556	2 Feb 1956	Menetelmä aminopiperidiini-2,6-dionen valmistamiseksi	
India	56475	3 Feb 1956	Process of preparing novel products of the Amino-Piperidine-2,6-Dione Series	Inventors not named
East Germany	14576	4 Feb 1956	Verfahren zur Herstellung von Amino-piperidin-2,6-dionen	Keller, Kunz

Country	No.	Date of application	Title	Notes
Australia	209532	7 Feb 1956	Processes of preparing novel products of the Amino-Piperidine-2,6-Dione Series	Keller, Kunz
Denmark	55956	15 Feb 1956	Fremgangsmåde til fremstilling af amino-piperidin-2,6-dionforbindelser	
Belgium	548074	24 May 1956	Procédé de fabrication d'amino-pipéridine-2,6-diones	Inventors not named
West Germany	1093364	11 Jun 1956	Verfahren zur Herstellung von Derivaten von Amino-piperidin-2,6-dionen	Inventors not named; patent references Austrian patent AT 174,909 for glutethimide (Doriden).
South Africa	Application no.: 1956/02068	27 Jul 1956	New products of the amino piperidine-2-6 dione and process of preparing the same	Keller, Kunz
Canada	585464	Not recorded	Products of the Amino-Piperidine-2,6-Dione Series and process thereof	Keller, Kunz Issue date 20 Oct 1959
Cyprus	19960	31 May 1960	Novel products of the Amino-Piperidine-2,6-Dione Series	
Malaysia	3360	N/A (published 31 Dec 1960)	Novel products of the Amino-Piperidine-2,6-Dione Series	Inventors not named

Descriptions of effects – first five thalidomide patents

Germany 1074584 Switzerland 336826	UK 768821 USA 2830991	France 1164512
Die Produkte verursachen eine stark ausgeprägte Minderung der Motilität, d. H. Des Bewegungstriebes, bei sehr geringer Toxizität; sie konnen allgemein zur 'Zentraldämpfung', z. B. Zur Behandliung von vegetativen Dystonien, eingesetzt warden. Die substanzen besitzen keine peripher lähmenden, curareatigen Wirkungen ... **(Switzerland only):** Darüber hinaus haben die Verbindungen gewisse spasmolytische und Antihistamin-Wirkungen. In größeren Mengen verabreicht, wirken die neuen Verbindungen, besonders das 3-Phthalimido-2,6-dioxopiperidin, als Schlafmittel	The products of the invention possess valuable therapeutic properties. They cause a strongly pronounced lowering of the motility, i.e. the phenomenon of motion, and have a very low toxicity. They may be generally employed for 'central attenuation' (vegetative dystonia). The products of the invention do not have any peripherally paralysing curare-like effects. In addition, the compounds have certain spasmolytic and antihistaminic effects. Dispensed in larger quantities, the products of the invention, and particularly 3-phthalimido-2,6-dioxopiperidine are effective as soporifics...	Les produits obtenus par al mise en oeuvre du présent procédé possèdent des propriétés thérapeutiques intéressantes. Ils provoquent une diminution très prononcée de la motilité et possèdent une très faible toxicité. Ils peuvent d'une façon générale servir pour la dystonie neuro-végétative. Ces composés n'exercent aucun effet de paralysiie périphérique analogue à celui du curare, et ils possèdent certaines propriétés anti-spasmodiques et antihistaminiques. A doses plus importantes, ils agissent comme hypnotiques, en particulier le 3-phthalimido-2,6-dioxopiperidine.

Appendix 2

Piperidine derivative patents 1927 – 1953

Date	Registration	Notes	Effects
1927 12 Jan	USA 1,752,617 for Winthrop Chemical Company Inc	*Werner Schulemann,* Fritz Schonhofer, and August Winkler of Elberfeld (Bayer); process for the aminoalkylation of amines; (five examples given showing piperidine base molecule), and referencing German patents 52,228; 52,229; and 52,230 (all 1925) and US patent 1,747,521; filed in Germany Jan 25 1927	Pharmaceutical products; blue dye shades
1931 20 Jun	UK 382,922 for I G Farbenindustrie	'Manufacture of a Sulphonic Acid of Piperidine or of an Alkyl Homologue of Piperidine'	Pharmaceutical ly active products
1935 18 Jun	Germany 634284 for Hoffman LaRoche	2-4 Dioxo-piperidine	Strong hypnotic
1935 6 Sep	Germany 637875 for Hoffman LaRoche	2-4 Dioxo-piperidine	Hypnotic activity in smallest doses
1935 29 Aug	Germany 634285 for Hoffman LaRoche	2-4 Dioxo-piperidine	Strong hypnotic
1935 5 Sep	Germany 637385 for Hoffman LaRoche	2-4 Dioxo-piperidine	Strong hypnotic
1937 8 Aug	Germany 679281 for Hoffman LaRoche	Piperidines ("Piperidinverbidungen") Dr. Otto Eisleb, Frankfurt, Main	Therapeutics, spasmolytic and analgesic
1939 31 Mar	Germany 713746 for I G Farbenindustrie	4-Arylpiperidyl-4-ketonen Dr. Otto Eisleb, Hofheim, Taunus	Spasmolytic and analgesic, low toxicity

Date	Registration	Notes	Effects
1941 15 Jan	Germany 872 045 for Schering AG	Dr. Rudolf Tschesche, Berlin-Wilmersdorf, Dr. Hermann Fox, Berlin-Frohnau und Dr. Karl Junkmann, Berlin. Verfahren zur Herstellung von Abkommlingen des 4-Oxypiperidins.	Spasmolytic
1942 19 May	Germany 752 755 for I G Farbenindustrie	Dr. Otto Eisleb, Hofheim (Taunus) A G; Verfahren zur Herstellung von 1-Alkyl-4-(m-oxyphenyl)-piperidinverbindungen	Good Spasmolytic and painkiller
1942 23 Jun	Germany 748800 for I G Farbenindustrie	1-Aryl-piperidin-4-carbonsäurederivaten Dr. Otto Eisleb, Hofheim, Taunus	Therapeutics
1942 29 Dec	Germany 897561 for Hoechst	4-Aryl-N-Alkyl-piperidin-4-carbonsäurenitrilen und -estern Dr. Gustav Erhardt, Frankfurt, Main	Spasmolytic, analgesic, low toxicity
1944 24 Aug	US 2506605 for Geigy	1-Alkyl-4-hydroxy-piperidine esters of alkyl substituted acetic acids Henry Martin, Alfred Margot, Basel Switzerland	Strong effect on parasympatholytic nervous system like atropine, but reduced toxicity
1944 1 Sep	UK 595631 for Hoffman LaRoche, New Jersey	Improvements – Piperidine Derivatives 7 example processes	Spasmolytic 5 times stronger than papaverine (opium alkaloid) same toxicity level
1946 24 Jan	UK 646,198 for Winthrop Stearns	'Improvements in or relating to the Preparation of Antispasmodic agents'; includes *3 piperidine derivatives*	Antispasmodic
1948 12 Jun	Austria 256347 for Hoffman LaRoche	1,3,3,-trimethyl 2-4 Dioxo piperidine	Antiepileptic
1948 18 May	Austria 167093 for Hoffman LaRoche	1,3,3,-trimethyl 2-4 Dioxo piperidine	Antiepileptic

Date	Registration	Notes	Effects
1949 28 Jan	USA 2,680,115 for Winthrop Stearns	'Substituted Tertiary-Aminoalkyl Carbinols' Arlo Wayne Ruddy, Albany NY; Theodore J. Becker, deceased, late of Albany, NY, by Maurice L. Tainter, administrator, Albany NY, listing *7 piperidine derivatives*	Antispasmodic agents, compared with atropine
1949 28 Jan	USA 2,662,886 for Winthrop Stearns	'Substituted Phenylpropylamines' Arlo Wayne Ruddy, Morristown NJ; Theodore J. Becker, deceased, late of Delmar, NY, by Maurice L. Tainter, listing *21 piperidine derivatives*	Antispasmodic agents, compared with atropine
1950 7 Jul	Austria 172933 for CIBA	'Verfahren zur Herstellung neuer Dioxopiperidine'. (2,6-dioxo-piperidine compound very similar to thalidomide)	Excellent parasympatholytic
1951 3 Jul	Germany 927,330 (Austrian: 174909 13 Feb 1951) for CIBA	Dr. Karl Hoffmann, Binningen und Dr. Eugen Tagmann, Basel (Schweiz); Aktiengesellschaft, Basel (Schweiz): Verfahren zur Herstellung neuer Dioxopiperidine. (2,6-dioxo-piperidine compound very similar to thalidomide)	Excellent parasympatholytic
1951 13 Feb	Germany 950 193 for CIBA	Dr. Karl Hoffmann, Binningen, und Dr. Eugen Tagmann, 'Verfahren zur Herstellungen neuer Dioxopiperidine'. Glutethimide; main trade name Doriden; a 2,6-dioxo-piperidine	Excellent anticonvulsive agent
1951 3 Jul	Germany 927330 for CIBA	New Dioxopiperidine Dr. Karl Hoffman, Dr. Eugen Tagmann Related to Doriden	Anticonvulsive
1951 17 Aug	USA 2,739,968 for Schering Corporation	Nathan Sperber, Bloomfield, NJ; Frank J. Viullani, Brooklyn, NY; and Dominic Papa, Bloomfield, NJ; 'Substituted Piperidines', a total of *134 piperidines*	All having 'antihistaminic, antispasmodic, antiacetylcholine and analgesic activity'

Date	Registration	Notes	Effects
1951 14 Nov	UK 740,689 for Schering Corporation	Substituted Piperidines, a further *97 piperidines*	All having 'antihistaminic, antispasmodic, antiacetylcholine and analgesic activity'
1952 26 Feb	Switzerland 309336 for CIBA	New Oxypiperidin	Very anticonvulsive
1953 24 Mar	Germany 1,003,209 for BASF, Ludwigshafen	Dr. Walter Reppe, Dr. Heinrich Pasedach, Dr. Erich Dreher, Dr. August Amann; a piperidine derivative very close in type to thalidomide	Spasmolytic, effective with Parkinson's disease
1953 22 Dec	Switzerland 326774 for CIBA	New Piperidine Dr. Karl Hoffman, Dr. Jules Heer, Dr. Ernst Sury, Dr. Ernst Urech	Central nervous system effect

Appendix 3

Grünenthal patents from thalidomide analogue and derivative research programme 1965-2001

Patent no.	Application date	Applications, details	No. of items
DE 1 545 672	8 May 1965	Dikarbonsäureimidderivative und Verfahren zu ihrer Herstellung. Inventors: Ernst Frankus; *Heinrich Mückter.* Anti-tumour	16
UK 1 075 420	9 May 1966 (Germany 8 May 1965)	Cyclic Imide Compounds and a process for their production Anti-tumour, transplant tissue survival (immunosuppressive), leprous diseases, auto-immune diseases, endocrine and sedative effects	21
DE 1 545 706	12 Oct 1965	Dicarbonsäureimidderivative und Verfahren zu ihrer Herstellung. Inventors: Ernst Frankus; *Heinrich Mückter.* Anti-tumour	3
DE 1 545 707	13 Oct 1965	Verfahren zur Herstellung von Dikarbonsäureimidderivativen Inventors: Ernst Frankus; *Heinrich Mückter;* Horst Böhlke. Anti-tumour	9
AU 260240	15 Oct 1965	Verfahren zur Herstellung von neuen Dikarbonsäureimidderivativen, sowie Salzen dieser Verbindungen Anti-tumour	38
DE 1 670 391	12 Oct 1966	Dikarbonsäureimidderivative und Verfahren zu ihrer Herstellung. Inventors: Ernst Frankus; *Heinrich Mückter;* Franz Otto. Anti-tumour	49
DE 1 670 443	1 Jul 1967	Phthalimidinderivate und Verfahren zur Herstellung Inventors: Ivars Graudums; *Heinrich Mückter;* Ernst Frankus; Sedative, immunosuppressive	9

Patent no.	Application date	Applications, details	No. of items
DE 2 210 166	3 Mar 1972	Neue Lactame und Verfahren zu ihrer Herstellung Inventors: Ivars Graudums; *Heinrich Mückter;* Ernst Frankus; Human & animal hypnotic, leprosy reaction (ENL), immunosuppressive, anti-tumour	10
DE 2 329 308	8 Jun 1973	Neue Lactame Inventors: Ivars Graudums; *Heinrich Mückter;* Ernst Frankus; Human & animal hypnotic, leprosy reaction, immunosuppressive, anti-tumour	5
DE 2 329 309	8 Jun 1973	Verfahren zur Herstellung von neuen Lactamen Inventors: Ivars Graudums; *Heinrich Mückter;* Ernst Frankus; Development of DE 2329308	1
DE 2 460 304	20 Dec 1974	1-n-Propyl-4-phthalimido-piperidin-2,6-dion, Verfahren zu seiner Herstellung und dieses enthaltende Arzneimittel Inventors: Ernst Frankus; *Heinrich Mückter;* Anti-tumour	10
DE 3 048 663	23 Dec 1980	Neue Lactamverbindungen, diese Arzneimittel und Verfahren zur Herstellung dieser Verbindungen und Arzneimittel Inventors: Ivars Graudums; Elmar Friedrichs Human and animal hypnotic, narcotic effect	23
DE 3 244 954	4 Dec 1982	Verfahren zur Herstellung von 3-(o-Sulfobenzoesäureimido)-piperidin-2-onen und neue Ausgangs- bzw. Zwischenprodukte für dieses Verfahren Inventor: Ivars Graudums; Pharmacological effect	4
DE 4 211 812	8 Apr 1992	Neue Thalidomidderivate, ein Verfahren zu deren Herstellung sowie die Verwendung derselben in Arzneimitteln Inventors: Kurt Eger; Gerhard Ehninger, Alfred Stuhler Intestinal lesions, Graft vs Host disease (immune system), immunosuppressive, immunomodulatory	5

Patent no.	Application date	Applications, details	No. of items
DE 4 422 237	24 Jun 1994	Verwendung von Lactamverbindungen als pharmazeutische Wirkstoffe Inventors: Horst Böhlke; Michael Finkam; Johannes Schneider; Oswald Zimmer; Kai Zwingenberger TNF- α inhibitor (anti-tumour), Graft vs Host disease, Behçet's (oral-genital ulcers), Lupus, Rheumatoid Arthritis	9
DE 19 613 976	9 Apr 1996	Thalidomid-Prodrugs mit immunomodulatorischer Wirkung Inventors: Johannes Schneider; Werner Winter; Stephan Wnendt; Kai Zwingenberger; Kurt Eger; Michaela Akerman TNF- α inhibitor, Graft vs Host disease, Multiple Sclerosis, Aphthoser stomatitis (ulcers), Morbus Boeck (lung disease), Behçet's, Lupus, Rheumatoid Arthritis, Pyoderma gangranosum	9
DE 19 703 763	1 Feb 1997	Thalidomidanalogue Verbindungen aus der Klasswe der Piperidin-2,6-Dione Inventors: Oswald Zimmer; Werner Winter; Stephan Wnendt; Kurt Eger; Uwe Teibert TNF- α inhibitor, Graft vs Host disease, Multiple Sclerosis, ENL, Aphthoser stomatitis, Morbus Boeck, Lupus, Rheumatoid Arthritis, Behçet's, Pyoderma gangranosum	4
DE 19 743 968	6 Oct 1997	Intravenöse Applikationsform von Thalidomid zur Therapie immunologischer Erkrankungen Inventors: Sven Björkman; Peter Höglund; Tommy Eriksson Immunosuppression, Lupus, Pyoderma gangranosum, HIV (2 apps), orogenital ulcers, Behçet's	2
DE 198 43 793	24 Sep 1998	Substituierte Benzamide Inventors: Tieno Germann; Stefanie Frosch; Oswald Zimmer Rheumatiod Arthritis, Multiple Sclerosis, Diabetes, Psoriasis	3

Patent no.	Application date	Applications, details	No. of items
DE 19 914 621	31 Mar 1999	Die folgenden Angaben sind den vom Anmelder eingrechten Unterlagen entnommen Inventors: Tieno Germann; Heinrich Kugelmann Haematology-Oncology applications generally, TNF- α inhibitor, Graft vs Host disease, HIV, Multiple Sclerosis, Aphthous ulcers, Lupus, Behçet's, Pyoderma gangranosum, urogenital ulcers	1
DE 19 957 341	29 Nov 1999	Kombinationspräparat enthaldend eine Thalidomidverbindung und einen Phosphodiesterase Typ IV Inhibitor Inventors: Stefanie Frosch; Tieno Germann Immunomodulatory, Autoimmune disease, TNF- α inhibitor, Rheumatoid Arthritis, Multiple Sclerosis, ENL, Lupus, Behçet's, Allergic Encephalomyelitis, Diabetes	7
DE 10 002 509	21 Jan 2000	Substituierte Glutarimide Inventors: Tieno Germann; Stefanie Frosch; Erik Wade; Helmut Buschmann; Oswald Zimmer Autoimmune disease, immunoregulatory, Rheumatoid Arthritis, Multiple Sclerosis, Diabetes	8
DE 10 013 499	20 Mar 2000	Substituierte Benzamide Inventors: Stefanie Frosch; Tieno Germann; Oswald Zimmer Autoimmune disease, immunoregulatory, Rheumatoid Arthritis, Multiple Sclerosis, Diabetes	2
DE 10 163 595	21 Dec 2001	In 3-Position heterocyclisch substituierte Piperidin-2,6-dione Inventors: Helmut Buschmann; Stefanie Frosch; Tieno Germann; Oswald Zimmer Immunomodulatory, ENL, Oral ulcers, Immunosuppressive, tumour-reducing, Multiple Myeloma	1

Thalidomide anti-cancer patents with Grünenthal scientists Professor Dr. Kurt Eger and Dr. Uwe Teubert listed as inventors

GRÜNENTHAL

Patent no.	Date	Inventors Include:	Notes
DE 42 11 812	8 Apr 1992	Prof. Kurt Eger	Details above
DE 196 13 976	9 Apr 1996	Prof. Kurt Eger	Details above
DE 197 03 763	1 Feb 1997	Prof. Kurt Eger Uwe Teubert	Details above

US GOVERNMENT

Patent no.	Date	Inventors Include:	Notes
US Patent application publication 2004/0077685	27 Feb 2001	Prof. Kurt Eger Uwe Teubert (2nd & 3rd names)	Analogs of Thalidomide as potential anti-angiogenesis inhibitors
US 7,320 991	26 Feb 2002	Prof. Kurt Eger Uwe Teubert (2nd & 3rd names)	Analogs of Thalidomide as potential anti-angiogenesis inhibitors
CA 2 439 410	26 Feb 2002	Prof. Kurt Eger Uwe Teubert (2nd & 3rd names)	Analogs of Thalidomide as potential anti-angiogenesis inhibitors
US Patent application publication 2007/0293519	19 Jul 2007	Prof. Kurt Eger Uwe Teubert (2nd & 3rd names)	Analogs of Thalidomide as potential anti-angiogenesis inhibitors

Appendix 4

Grünenthal thalidomide trade name registrations in Latin America 1958-1999

Application Date	Product	Country	Reg. No.
01/01/1958	Softenon	Venezuela	1958-009390
01/01/1959	Peracon	Venezuela	1959-013155
21/05/1973	Enterosediv	Brazil	006207820
26/12/1978	Softenon	Colombia	92 14187 5
25/01/1979	Softenon	Chile	219596
18/01/1980	Softenon	Argentina	956055
05/03/1980	Softenil	Colombia	92 150310 B
05/03/1980	Enterosediv	Colombia	92 150310 A
28/05/1982	Softenon	Brazil	810863162
30/09/1983	Softenon	Colombia	92 194725 5
23/01/1998	Enterosediv	Argentina	233644
30/01/1998	Enterosediv	Venezuela	1998-001587
07/10/1998	Enterosediv	Chile	523602
05/11/1999	Talidomida Cassara	Argentina	38556

Index

U

V

W